MEDICINAL PLANTS OF INDIA

By

Professor Rasheeduz Zafar
M. Pharm., Ph.D.
Dean Faculty of Pharmacy
Head of the Dept. of Pharmacognosy Phytochemistry
Faculty of Pharmacy
Hamdard University
New Delhi

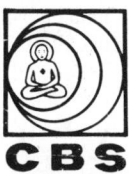

CBS

CBS Publishers & Distributors Pvt. Ltd.

New Delhi • Bengaluru • Chennai • Kochi • Kolkata • Mumbai
Hyderabad • Nagpur • Patna • Pune • Vijayawada

ISBN: 81-239-0277-8

First Edition: 1994
Reprint: 1998, 2000, 2002, 2004, 2009,
        2011, 2014, 2017, 2019

Published by **Satish Kumar Jain** and produced by **Varun Jain** for
CBS Publishers & Distributors Pvt. Ltd.,
4819/XI Prahlad Street, 24 Ansari Road, Daryaganj, New Delhi - 110002
delhi@cbspd.com, cbspubs@airtelmail.in • www.cbspd.com
Ph.: 23289259, 23266861, 23266867 • Fax: 011-23243014

Corporate Office: 204 FIE, Industrial Area, Patparganj, Delhi - 110 092
Ph: 49344934 • Fax: 011-49344935
E-mail: publishing@cbspd.com • publicity@cbspd.com

Branches:
• *Bengaluru:* 2975, 17th Cross, K.R. Road, Bansankari 2nd Stage,
  Bengaluru - 70 • Ph: +91-80-26771678/79 • Fax: +91-80-26771680
  E-mail: cbsbng@gmail.com, bangalore@cbspd.com
• *Chennai:* No. 7, Subbaraya Street, Shenoy Nagar, Chennai - 600030
  Ph: +91-44-26681266, 26680620 • Fax: +91-44-42032115
  E-mail: chennai@cbspd.com
• *Kochi:* Ashana House, 39/1904, A.M. Thomas Road, Valanjambalam,
  Ernakulum, Kochi • Ph: +91-484-4059061-65
  Fax: +91-484-4059065 • E-mail: cochin@cbspd.com
• *Kolkata:* 6-B, Ground Floor, Rameshwar Shaw Road, Kolkata - 700014
  Ph: +91-33-22891126/7/8 • E-mail: kolkata@cbspd.com
• *Mumbai:* 83-C, Dr. E. Moses Road, Worli, Mumbai - 400018
  Ph: +91-9833017933, 022-24902340/41 • E-mail: mumbai@cbspd.com

Representatives:

• Hyderabad: 0-9885175004	• Nagpur: 0-9021734563
• Patna: 0-9334159340	• Pune: 0-9623451994
• Jharkhand: 0-9811541605	• Uttarakhand: 0-9716462459

Printed at:
J.S. Offset Printers, Delhi (India)

Preface

India has a vast and inexhaustible resource of drugs of plant origin and India can supply these drugs to many other countries. The systematic investigation of these drugs used in indigenous medicine on modern scientific lines was started more than thirty years ago and much has been accomplished during this short time. A number of important medicinal plants prescribed by the Vaids and Hakims have been carefully investigated from every point of view. Their chemical composition has been determined, the pharmacological action of the active principles worked out by animal experimentation and it is only by such a thorough enquiry that the real merits of these drugs have been proved.

In the present book, a review of the scientific work done on ten medicinal plants has been presented. I am sure that it will be helpful to the researcher and students. Besides the chemical and pharmacological data on these medicinal plants, tissue culture work has also been reviewed.

I am extremely thankful to my post-graduate students and research scholars who have helped me in collecting the data on the medicinal plants included in the book. I am extremely thankful to Janab Hakim Abdul Hamid Saheb, Chancellor Jamia Hamdard and Janab Mueed Saheb for their encouragement.

RASHEEDUZ ZAFAR

Contents

1
Achyranthes aspera Linn

A survey of scientific literature revealed that work on *Achyranthes aspera* Linn can be divided under following headings.
A) Ethnobotany
B) Pharmacognsy
C) Phytochemistry
D) Pharmacology

A) ETHNOBOTANY

Achyranthes aspera has been used as medicine from ancient times for treating a large number of diseases. Different parts of the plant have been used in different ways. The whole plant has been used as a remedy for a number of diseases. A decoction of the plant made by boiling the plant in water had been recommended (Nadkarni, 1976)[1] as a diuretic and is used in renal dropsy, and general anasarca. The juice of plant is used to dissipate corneal opacity and to stop bleeding of wounds, when applied locally. In Philippines the plant is used to dissipate corneal opacity and to relieve tooth ache, dysentery and bowel complaints (Watt 1963)[2]. Root of the plant is said to be useful for the treatment of pneumonia (Haerdi and Eingeborenon, 1964)[3] and is also considered mild astringent in bowel complaints (Quisumbing 1951)[4]. The root has been used (Chopra 1933)[5] as stomachic & digestant in India. Egypt & Australia. It is reported to be useful in the treatment of piles & as a diuretic in many parts of world. In Africa the root is chewed and applied to cuts to stop bleeding. The extract of root has been used to treat menstrual disorders (Singh, Palvi & Singh, 1981)[6] whereas the powder of root mixed with crushed snails is used to cure leprosy (Rao, 1981)[7]. The root has been used to treat dysentery by taking its mixture in water, (Wilson and Mariam, 1979)[8]. Rootpaste is considered to be an antifertility drug (Malhi and Trivedi, 1972)[9]. With cold water, a root paste is given to stop bleeding after abortion and also used for early delivery (Sahu, 1982)[10]. Leaf juice is useful in stomach-ache, bowel complaints, piles and skin eruptions etc. and in large doses to produce labour pain abortions (Nadkarni, 1979)[1]. The leaf is used as a remedy for boil and abscess (Watt, 1962)[2]. In Philippines the leaf is used as an emetic (Quisumbing, 1951)[4]. A paste of leaf with water is used is treat bites of poisonous insects, wasps and bee, etc. Fresh juice of leaves with opium is used typically to treat primary syphilitic sores whereas. fresh leaves ground into paste with jaggery or black pepper is used as antiperiodic especially in quatrain fever. Reponda Walker (1961)[11], mentioned the use of leaves to hasten the maturing of abscess and to extract thorn from the feet. A decoction of leaf is used for treating early stages of diarrhoea and dysentery. The seeds of the plant are used to treat snake bites, hydrophobia, and itching in East Indies (Watt & Breyer, 1962)[2] and in India (Nadkarni, 1976)[1]. In Philippines (Quisumbing, 1951)[4] the seeds are used as an emetic and also used as a brain tonic and in bleeding piles (Mishra, Bihari, 1969)[12] and as a tonic in winter (Bhandari, 1974)[13]. The whole plant is used as inhalation in acute chills, as food in famine and as snuff in Tswana (Africa), renal dropsy (George, 1974)[14] bronchial infections (Gopalachari and Dhar, 1958)[15]. Vomiting of blood (George, 1974)[14] & hemorrhoids. The plant is also used for pain in loins, blindness in cattle and rheumatism (Shankar 1979[16], Jain and Tarafdar, 1970)[17]. The ash of the plant is said to be useful in cough (Chopra, 1933[5], Watt and Breyer, 1964[2], Nadkarni, 1976)[1], pain in the chest and as antacid due to its high potash content. The plant is reported to possess antidiabetic and antirheumatic properties (El-Kheir and Salik, 1980)[18]. It is also used beneficially in abdominal tumors (Hartwell, 1976)[19].

B) PHARMACOGNOSY

Achyranthes aspera Linn. (Fig. 1.1) is an erect plant, 0.3-0.9 meters high; with stem stiff, not much branched, branches

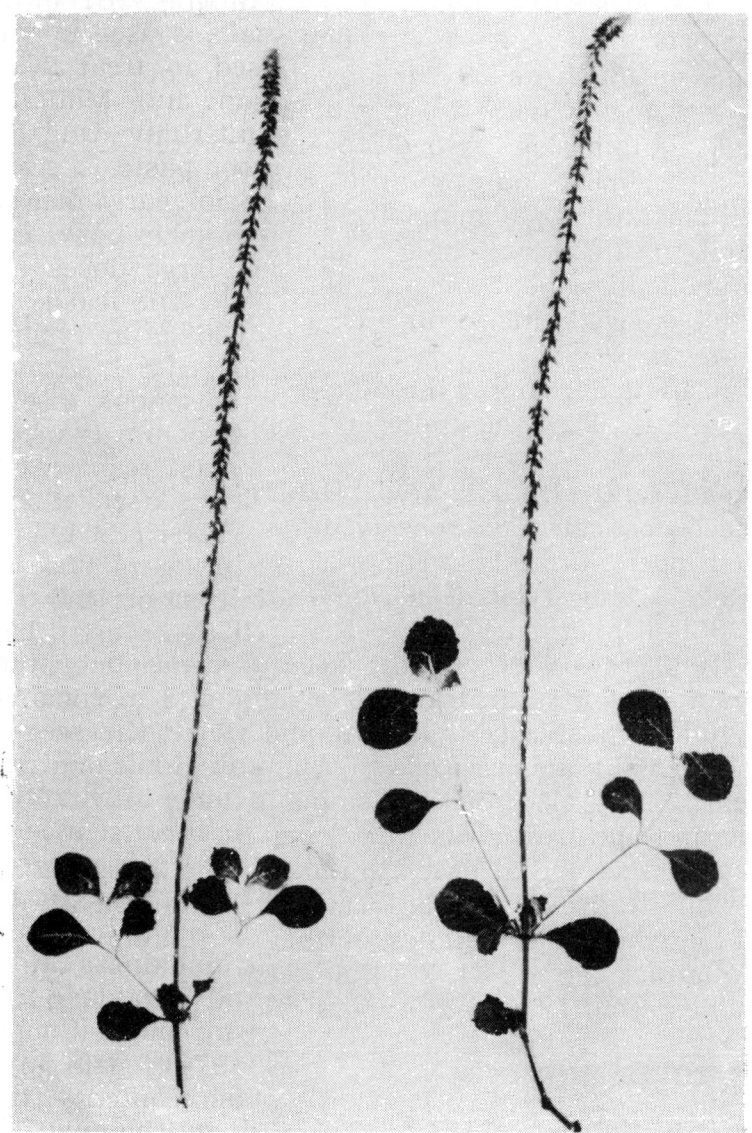

Fig. 1.1 Achyranthes aspera – Linn

terete or absolutely quadrangular, striate, pubescent; leaves few, usually thick, 3.8-6.3 x 22.5-4.5 cm, elliptic or obovate, sometimes nearly orbicular, usually rounded (rarely subactue) at the apex, finely and softly pubescent on both sides, entire, petiolate, petiole 6-20 mm long; flowers greenish white, numerous, stiffly deflexed against the woody pubescent rachis, in elongate terminal spikes which are at first short but soon lengthen, reaching, as much as 50 cm long in fruit; bracts 3 mm long, broadly ovate, acuminate, membranous, aristate, presistant; bracteoles 3 mm long, broadly ovate concave, with a spine as long as the blade, hard in fruit, falling off with the fruiting perianth; perianth 4-6 mm long, glabrous and shining, sepals subequal, ovate-oblong finely pointed, with narrow white membranous margins; stamens-5, staminodes truncate, fimbriate, utricle oblong-cylindric, truncate at the apex, rounded at the base, brown.

The plant is distributed throughout India, Baluchistan, Ceylon, Tropical Asia, Africa, Australia and America upto an altitude of 3000 ft.

Prasad and Bhatacharya (1961)[20] studied the plant pharmacognostically and observed an average stomatal index of 6.6 (Upper surface) and (Lower surface), Average Palisad Ratio 9.2, Average Vein Islet No 9, and average epidermal cell count 360 (Upper surface), and 455 (Lower surface), Paliwal et.al. (1980)[21] worked on the structure and development of stomata and reported the leaves to be amphistomatic with stomata mainly on lower surface and of anomocytic type. The epidermal cells showed sinuate cell walls to a limited extent and trichomes 2-3 celled. They also reported stomatal index as 33 (base), 30 (middle and apex), whereas the stomatal frequency (per sq.mm) was reported as 358 at base, 286 in the middle, and 261 at the apex of the leaf. Joshi, (1931)[22] and Dastur (1935)[23] worked on the primary vascular bundles of the plant from the antigenic point. Karnick et. al. (1976)[24] studied the effect of different lunar phases on the growth of plant.

C) PHYTOCHEMISTRY

In 1958, Gopalachari and Dhar isolated a saponin from the alcoholic extract of defatted seeds of *Achyranthes aspera* which was obtained as a light brown gummy mass. The saponin on acid hydrolysis gave a sapogenin-oleanolic acid and four sugars, which were identified by paper chromatography as glucose, galactose, xylose and rhamnose. Khastgir et.al. (1958)[26] also found oleanolic acid from seeds. Harihara & Rangaswami (1970)[27] studied in detail the saponin and found that the saponin was a mixture of two saponins, referred to as saponin A & saponin B. (The dimethyl derivative of saponin gave two spots when chromatographed). These saponins were on detailed chemical investigation found to be as saponin A=L-rhamnopyranosyl-(1-4)-β-D-(1-3)-oleanolic acid. Saponin B=β-D-Galactopyransyl (1-28)-ester of Saponin A. (Fig. 1.2)

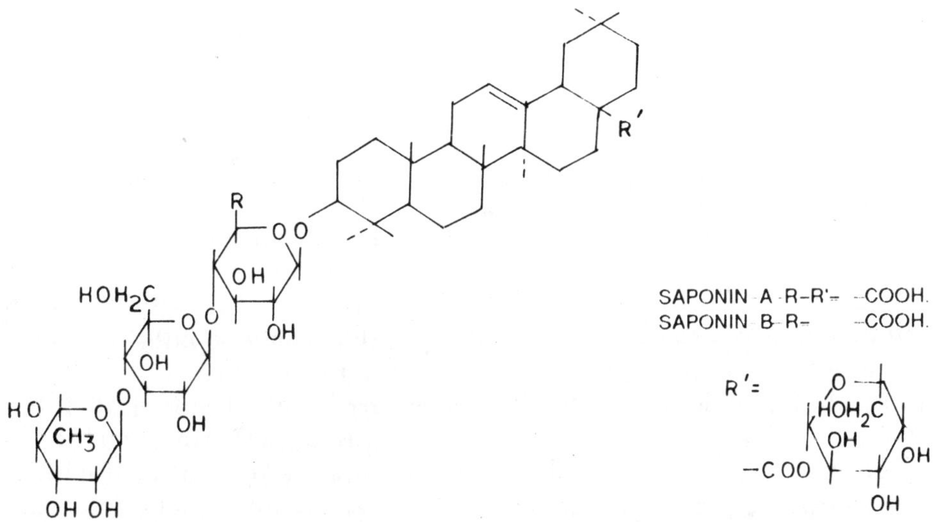

SAPONIN A R–R'= –COOH.
SAPONIN B R– –COOH.

Fig. 1.2 Structural Formula of Saponin A and B

Sheshadri, Batta and Rangaswami (1931)[28] have reported the presence of two new saponins in the unripe fruits. They are: (Fig. 1.3)

Khastgir & Sengupta (1958)[29] isolated a saponin from the root of the plant. On examination, oleanolic acid was found to be the aglycone of this saponin also. Sarkar and Rastogi (1960)[30] developed a method of separation and isolation of triterpenoid saponin by descending paper chromatography. They obtained four spots from Achyranthes saponins in two systems. The pet ether extract of seeds gave a fatty matter which was found to be a hydrocarbon with molecular formula $C_{31} H_{64}$ and appeared to be Hentriacontane (Parks, West and Naylor, 1946)[31]. Satyanarayana et.al. (1964)[32] analysed the seeds of the plant for their protein, amino acid, carbonydrate, iron, calcium & phosphorous content.

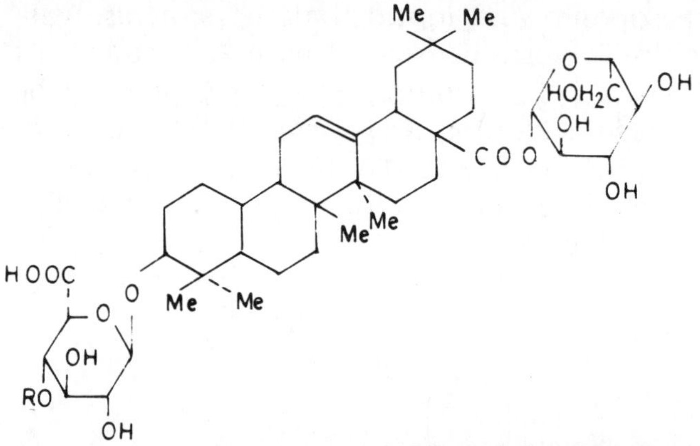

SAPONIN—C=R=L–Rhamnopyranosyl.
SAPONIN—d=R=L Rhamnopyranosyl–(1–4)–D–Glycopyranosyl.

Fig. 1.3 Structural Formula of Saponin C and D

Central Council for Research in Indian Medicine & Homoeopathy (1976)[33]. standardised the ash of the plant known commonly as Apamarga Kshara for its magnesium. sodium. potassium. calcium. iron. chloride. sulphate. and phosphate content. Anand Kumar *et.al.* (1982)[34] analysed the ash of the plant for the water soluble matter and minerals which included potassium. calcium. magnesuim. sodium. iron and ion of chloride. carbonate. sulphate and phosphate. Basu *et.al.* (1957)[35] subjected the whole plant to chemical analysis. they isolated a water soluble alkaloid which melted at 292-3°C (with decomp) its various derivatives were prepared which included hydrochloride (m.p.273°C). sulphate (m.p. 182-3°C). picrate (m.p.181°C) gold chloride complex (m.p. 199°C) bismuth iodide complex (m.p. 260°C) & reinicate (m.p. 160°C with decomp). The base was hygroscopic sand found to contain one molecule of water of crystallization. Its molecular formula was found to be $C_6 H_{11} NO_2 . H_2O$. Its is known as *Achyranthine* and is a Betaine derivative of N-Methyl pyrrolidine-3-carboxylic acid (Basu 1957)[35]. They also isolated another base which was water insoluble. chloroform soluble and alkaloidal in nature. Because of low yields it could not be further worked out for structure analysis. This base was light yellow. and resinous in nature which could not be crystallized. Besides there two alkaloids. they also obtained large quantities of inorganic salts consisting chiefly of potassium chloride. They further reported the presence of reducing sugars and disaccharides in the plant.

Kapoor & Singh (1966)[36] isolated another water soluble base which on elemental analysis corresponded to $C_5 H_{11} NO_2$ and compared with betaine on the basis of physical and chemical properties and I.R. spectra. Kapoor & Singh (1967)[37] showed that chloroform soluble basic fraction isolated by Basu *etal.* (1957)[35] was not chromatographicaslly homogenous as it gave two spots when paper chromatographed. Farooq Hasan (1962)[38] reported the presence of vitamin C in the plant (29 mg vitamin-C/100 gm whole plant). Ikram and Islam (1963)[39] reported the absence of alkaloids in the leaves and stem of *Achyranthes aspera*.

Banerjee and Chadha (1970)[40] isolated from the methanolic extract of root a compound-ecdysterone, a colourless crystelline compound with a molecular formula $C_{24}H_{44}O_7$ and M.P > 237°-239°C. Hiroshi *et.al.* (1971[41], 1975)[42] observed the presence of inokosterone and ecdysterone in callus and tissue culture of Achyranthes on White's media containing 10% coconut milk and 1 ppm 2. 4-D. In 1978 Shekhawat *et.al.*[43] correlated the increased carbohydrate, phendperoxidase, and polyphenol oxidase decreased during maturation but in gall tissues, the activity of peroxidase and polyphenol oxidase increased in old tissues. In healthy tissues, the IAA-oxidase activity is reduced with age but reverse was the case for gall tissues. Purohit *et.al.* (1980)[44] studied the enzyme levels in normal and white rust (Albugo biti) infected leaves and studied the involvement of this enzyme with the stage of infection. It was observed that with the severity of infection, there was a gradual increase in peroxidase and IAA-oxidase activity. Decreased total O-dihydroxy phenol with increased polyphenol oxidase activity was observed in infected leaves when compared with healthy leaves. Gradual increase in enzymatic activity with decreased phenolics showed a state of catabolism induced by pathogenesis.

D) PHARMACOLOGY

The plant has been tested for various pharmacological properties.

a) ABORTIFACIENT ACTIVITY

Basu *et.al.* (1957)[35] observed that 1% solution of achyranthine caused immediate contractions of both gravid & non-gravid uterus. Kapoor and Singh (1967)[37] found that chloroform soluble, water isoluble alkaloidal portion did not have any direct effect on the uterine muscle but it checked the spasms produced by 0.2 ug/ml acetyl choline chloride.

Pakrashi *et.al.* (1975)[45] found significant antifertility effect in benzene extract of stem bark of the plant. Pakrashi and Bhattacharya (1977)[46], observed that the benzene fraction of benzene extract of the plant in a single dose of 50 mg per kg body weight showed cent percent abortifacient activity in rabbit. The drug was neither estrogenic, nor antiesstrogenic or androgenic in mice. Abortion may not be due to the deficiency in prolactin, growth hormones or pituitary gonadotropins. The drug is non toxic & non teratogenic.

b) CARDIOVASCULAR ACTIVITY

In 1957 Basu *et.al.*[35] observed that Achyranthine at the dose levels of 0.4, 2 & 3 ml of 1 in 50 solution had no affect on blood pressure of ether anesthetized dog whereas chloroform soluble base (rendered soluble in water in the form of hydrochloride) caused slight depression of blow-pressure at the dose levels of 1 & 2 ml of 1% solution but this effect was of short duration. Aqueous extract of crude drug (0.1 ml 1:1 solution) showed some fall in amplitude of contractions of pithed from heart, thus showing a depresent action. Crude aqueous extract produced a definite constriction of blood vassels of frog as evidenced by reduction in perfussion rate by 32% at a dose level of 1 ml of 1:1 extract and 45.5% at a dose level of 2ml 1:1 extract. Kapoor and Singh (1966)[36] reported that chloroform soluble base increased the blood-pressure and the amplitude of cardiac contractions in anesthetized dog at the dose level of 10 mgkg body weight. In case of isolated guinea pig heart, Kapoor and Singh observed that 500 mcg of alkaloid decreased the rate of cardiac contractions but increased the amplitude substantially and also increased the coronary overflow. 1 mg dose of alkaloid caused initial depression in which both the rate and amplitude decreased which was followed by a little increase in the rate and almost 100% increased in the amplitude. but there was no change in the outflow. In 1970 Neogi *et.al.*[47] reported that

Achyranthine. a water alkaloid obtained from the plant reduced the heart rate and blood-pressure and dilated the blood vesseles in frog and dog. Gupta. Ram and Bhagwat (1972)[48] observed that a mixture of saponins isolated from the seeds of the plant caused a significant increase in force of contractions of isolated frog heart. guinea pig heart and rabbit heart. The stimulant effect of lower doses (1-50 mg) of saponin appeared to be exerted indirectly. as it was blocked by pronethelol and partly by mepyramine. The effect of higher doses appeared to be of direct nature and is not blocked by pronetholol. In addition the saponin increased the tone of heart rendered hypodynamic and also increased the force of contractions of failing papillary muscle. The effect was quick in onset and shorter in duration in comparison to that exerted by digoxin. Ram *et.al.* (1971)[49] studied the effect of saponin of *A.aspera* on the phosphorylase activity of rat heart. before and after perfusion of saponin and adrenalin.

c) EFFECTS ON URINARY TRACT

Kapoor and Singh (1967)[37] reported a little antidiuretic activity in the chloroform soluble basic fraction (alkaloid) at 150 mg per kg. body weight of albino rats. Gupta. Ram and Tripathi(1973)[50] reported the diuretic action of seed sponin of A. aspera. It was shown that the doses between 10-20 mg per kg. body weight given intramuscularly to rats caused a significant increase in urine output after 2.6 and 24 hrs. as compared to untreated control. The diuretic effect of 10 mg per kg. body weight dose of saponin was found to be optimum as there was no increase in urine output on increasing the dose of saponin. Significant increase in urine output was also observed in rats given 5-10 mg per kg body weight orally. and the effect was comparable to that observed with 10 mg per kg. body weight oral dose of acetazolamide. The diuretic effect of saponin. like that of acetaxolsamide. was also found to be associated with significant increase in excretion of sodium and potassium in the urine. *Achyranthes aspera* extract is one of the ingredients of cystone table which are widely being used to treat urinary tract infections and stones in the urinary tract (Ghosh Gupta, Chatterjee and Ghoshal, 1980)[51].

d) ANTIBACTERIAL & ANTIFUNGAL ACTIVITY

George *et.al.* (1947)[14] showed antibacterial activity of alcoholic and aqueous extracts of leaf of *A.aspera* against *E. coli*, and *S.aureus*. Basu, Neogi and Srivastava (1957)[52] observed the antibacterial activity of achyranthine and aqueous extract of plant against *S.aureus, Streptococcus haemolyticus,* and *Bacillus.* They also observed the anthelmintic activity of achyranthine and aqueous extract against earthworm. According to them the aqueous extract was more toxic to earth worm than the Achyranthiner, probably due to its high content of inorganic salts. Dhar *et.al.* (1968)[53] tested the plant extract for the following activities:

Antibacterial activity against :-

1) Gram Positive Organisms - *B.subtilis, Staphylococcus aureus.*

2) Gram Negative Organisms - *E. coli & S. typhi.*

3) Acid Fast Strain - *Mycobacterium tuberculosis*

Antifungal activity against various fungi like *Candida albicans, Aspergillus niger,* etc.

Antiprotozoal activity against *Entamoeba histolytica, Plasmodium bergheir* etc. and antiviral activity.

They did not find andy of the above mentioned activities to an appreciable extent.

Khurana, Paul and Bhargawe (1970)[54] found that crude leaf extract of the plant inhibits the activities of Mild-mosaic (MM), Distortion Ring spot (DR) and Ring Spot (RS) viruses of papaya *(Carica papaya).* Ikram and Haq (1980)[55] found the antibacterial activity of stem and leaf extract against *E. Coli, B. subtilis, Shigella dysenteriae* and *S. typhi.*

e) JUVENILE ACTIVITY

Rajendran and Gopalan (1978)[56] took pet. ether extract of whole plant and dried it, then they dissolved the residue in acetone and applied typically to larvae of *Dysdercus cingulatus* (Order Hemiptera, Family Pyrrhocoridae). It resulted in normal adults with fully formed wings which completely cover the abdomen. No black pigments on the abdominal tergum were observed and tarsi were 3-segmented. This observation indicated 100% juvenile activity.

The plant contains photoecdysones, namely ecdysterone and inokosterone (Banerjee *et.al.* 1971)[57]. Masatoshi et.al. (1967)[58] reported that 0.005-0.5 mcg dose of ecdysterone or 0.05-0.5 mcg dose of inokosterone when injected into housefly *(Meusca domestica)* larvae, induced pupations in 55% or more larie. 1 mcg dose of ecdysterone or Inokosterone when injected to duerpupae of silk worm *(Bombyx mori)* produced normal moths in 14-20 days after injection in more that 90% of months. 10 mcg of either substance when injected, all pupae became pupaladult mixtures without scales and scale hairs. On housefly, ecdysterone was found to be slightly more active that inokosterone (Takemoto *et.al.* 1967)[59]. Ecdysterone has a potential use a chemosterilant (Robins *et.al.* (1968)[60]. It stimulates protein synthesis in insects (Sekeris, Lang & Karlson, 1965)[61] and in mammals (Otaka *et.al.* 1980)[62].

f) MISCELLANEOUS ACTIONS

In 1968 Dhar *et.al.*[53]. reported a significant antidiabetic (hypoglycemic) activity in plant extract in albino rats. Kapoor and Singh (1967)[37] reported spasmolytic activity of chloroform soluble alkaloidal fractions, against various spasmogens (including acetyl choline chloride, histamine phosphate & $BaCl_2$) on intestine, and uterine muscle. Neogi, Rathor, and Garg (1970)[47] reported some spasmogenic activity of achyranthine on rectus abdominis muscle. It's spasmogenic activity at a dose level of 0.5 mg/ml was less than that of acetyl choline (0.1 mg/ml) but was not blocked by d-tubocuraine indicating that it was not mediated through cholinergic nerve endings. Srivastava (1966)[63] claimed that lepromaous type of leprosy can be cured in 10 days by a medicine made from an extract of fresh leaves of A.aspera. The bhasma of *Achyranthes aspera* was found to be useful in the treatment of bronchial asthma (Chayaralu, 1982)[64]. Mahaskar and Cauis (1931)[65] had found that plant offers no relief (symptomatic or systemic) used by ancient people and tribes. Saha Kalyanasundaram (1962)[66] claimed that the anthers of *Achyranthes aspera might* be responsible for seasonal allergy (hay fever, rhinitis etc.) in Pondicherry though the plant is entomophilous.

References

1. Nadkarni, K.M., *Indian Materia Medica*. I. 1976. Bombay Popular Prakashan. 21.
2. Watt, J.M., Breyer, M.G., *The Medicinal and Poisonous Plants of Southern and eastern Aftrica*, 1963, II Ed. E and S Livingst Ltd. Edinburgh and London.
3. Haerdi, F., Eingerborenon, D., *Acta Tropica Suppl*. 1964, 8 (1), 278.
4. Quisumbing, E., *Tech. Bull. Phillip. Dep. Agric. Nat. Res.* 1951, 16
5. Chopra, R.N., *Indigenous Drug Of India*. 1933. The Art. Press Calcutta., 230.
6. Singh, K.K., Palvi, S.K. Singh, H.B. *Ind. J. for.*, 1981, 4(2), 115.
7. Rao, R.T., *Econ. Bot.* 1981, 35(1), 4
8. Wilson, R.T., Mariam, W.G., *Econ Bot.* 1979, 33(1), 29.
9. Malhi, B.S., Trivedi, V.P., *Quert. J. Crude Drugs Res.*, 1972, 12(1), 1922.
10. Sahu, W.A., Sillens, R., *Les Plantes Utilesw du Gubun*, 1961, Paul Lechevalier, Paris, 132.
11. Rponda Walkar, A. and Sillens, R 1961 "Les Plantes utiles du Gabon", Paul Lechevalier, Paris.
12. Mishra, M.N., Bihari, R., *Labdev. J. Sci. Tech*, 1969 **7B**(3), 195
13. Bhandari, M.N., *Econ. Bot.*, 1974, **28**(1), 73.
14. George, M., *J. Sci Indust. Res.*, 1947, **6B**(3), 42.
15. Gopalachari, R., Dhar, M.L., *J. Sci. Indust. Res.*, **11B** (5), 209
16. Shankar, M.R., *Nagarjun*, 1979, **29**(1), 9.
17. Jain, S.K., Tarafdar, C.R., *Econ. Bot.*, **24**(3), 241.
18. El-Kheir, Y.M., Salik, M.H., *Fitoterpia*, 1980, **51**(3), 43.
19. Hartwell, J.L., *Lloydia*, 1970, **30**(4), 379.
20. Prasad, S. Bhattacharya, I.C., *J. Sci. Indust. Res.*, 1961, **20C**(8), 246.
21. Paliwal, G.S., Gupta, B.P., Males, C.B., *Ind. J. For.*, 1980, **3**(2), 135.
22. Joshi, A.C., *J. Ind. Bot. Soc.*, 1931, **10**, 1265.

23. Dastur, R.H., *Annals Bot. Soc.*, 1935, **39,** 539.
24. Karnic, C.R., Jopat, P.D., *Indian drug Pharm. Ind.*, 1976, **35**, 693
25. Gopalanchari, R., Dhar, M.L., *J.Sci. Indust. Res. (India),* 1985, **17**(B), 276
26. Khastgir, H., Sengupta, S.K., Sengupta, P., *J. Ind. Chem. Soc.*, 1958, **35**, 693.
27. Hariharan, V., Rangaswami, S., *Phytochem,* 1970, **9**(2), 379.
28. Sheshadri, V., Batta, A,K., Rangaswami, S., *Ind. J. Chem.*, 1981, **20B**(9), 773.
29. Khastgir, H., Sengupta, P., *J. Ind. Chem. Soc.,* 1958, **35**, 529.
30. Sarkar, B., Rastogi, R.P., *J. Sci. Indust. Res.*, 1960, **19B**(3), 106.
31. Parks G.S., West, J.J., Naylor, B.F., *J. Ame, Chem. Soc.,* 1946, **68**, 2524.
32. Satyanarayana, M.S., Sushila, B.A., Rao, A.N., Vijayraghwan, P.K., *J.Food. Sci. Tech.,* 1946, **1**(2), 26.
33. Central Council for Research in Indian Medicine & Homoeopathy, New Delhi. "Pharmaespecial Standard for Ayurvdedia Formulations P.17.
34. Anand Kumar, A., Thirugnanasambanatham, P., Rajendran, V., Murlidharan, K., Balasubramaniam, M., *J. Net. Integ. Med. Ass.* 1982, **24**(5), 141.
35. Basu, N.K., Sing, H.K., Aggarwal, O.P., *J. Proc. Inst. Chemists,* (India), 1957, **29**(1), 55.
36. Kapoor, V.K., Singh, H.K., *Ind. J. Chem,* 1966, **4**(10), 461.
37. Kapoor, V.K., Singh. H.K., *Ind. J. Pharm.,* 1967, **29**(10), 285.
38. Farooq Hasan, *Pakistan J. Sci. Res.,* 1962, **14**(1), 4.
39. Ikram, M., Islam, M., *Pakistan J. Sci. Indust. Res.,* 1963, **6**(1) 53.
40. Banerji, A., Chadha, M.S., *Phytochem.,* 1970, **9**(7), 1671.
41. Hiroshi, H., Hisanori, J., Takemoto, T., *Chem. Pharm. Bull.* 1971, **19**(2), 438.
42. Hiroshi, H., Hisanori, J., Takemoto, T., *Yakugaku Zasshi* 1975, **95**(5),581

43. Shekhawat, N.S., Ramawal, K.G., Arya, H.C., *Curr Sci,* 1978, **47**(20), 780.

44. Purohit, S., Bhattacharya, I.C., *J. Sci. Indust. Res.,* 1961, **20**C(8), 246.

45. Pakrashi, A., Mookerji, N., Basak, B., *J. Repord. Fert.,* 1975, **43**, 127.

46. Parkrashi, A., Bhattacharya, N, Ind. *J. Exp. Biol.,* 1977, **15**(10), 856

47. Neogi, N.C., Gar, R.D., Rathor, R.S., *Ind. J. Pharm.,* 1970, **32**(2),43

48. Gupta, S.S., Ram, A.K., Bhagwat, A.W., *Ind. J. Med, Res.,* 1972, **60**(3), 462.

49. Ram, A.K., Bhagwat, A.W., Gupta, S.S., *Ind. J. Physiol. Pharmacy.,* 1971, **15**(3),107.

50. Gupta, S.S., Ram A.K., Tripathi, R.M., *Ind. J. Pharmacol.,* 1972, **4**(4),4.

51. Ghosh, A., Sengupta, P., Chatterjee, S., Ghoshal, K.K., *Probe.* 1980, **19**(4),270.

52. Basu, N.K., Neogi, N.C., Srivastava, V.P., *J. Proc. Inst. Chem,* 1957, **29**(5), 161

53. Dhar, M.L., Dhar, M.M., Dhawan, B.N., Merhotru, B.N., Roy, C., *Ind. J. Exp. Bio.,* 1968, **5**(4), 232.

54. Khurana, L.M. Paul, S.M., Bhargawa, K.S., *J. App. Microbiol.,* 1970, **16**(3),225.

54. Ikram, M., Haq, I., Fitoterpia, 1980, 51(5), 231.

56. Rajendran, B., Gopalan, M., Ind. *J. Agri. Sci.,* 1978, **48**(5), 306.

57. Banerji, A., Chitalwar, G.J., Joshi, A.K., Chadha, M.S., *Phytochem,* 1971, **10**(9), 2225.

58. Masatoshi, K., Takemoto, T., Ogawa, S., Nishimoto, N., *J. Insect. Physiol,* 1967, **13**, (9), 1395.

59. Takemoto, T., Ogawa, S., Nishimoto, N., Mue, K., *Yakugaku Zasshi,* 1967, **87**(12), 1481.

60. Robins, W.E., Kaplanis, J.N., Thompson, T.J., Cohen, C.F., Joyner, S.C., *Science,* 1968, **161**, 1158,

61. Sekeris, C.E; Lang, N., Karlson, P., *J. Physiol Cheem.,* 1965, **36**, 341.

62. Otaka, T., Uchiyama, M., Okai, S., Takemoto, T., Hikino, H., Ogawa, S., Nishimoto, N., *Chem. Pharm. Bull. Japan,* 1980. **16**, 2426.

63. Srivastava, R.P., *Eastern Pharmacist*, 1966, **2**(100), 107.
64. Chayaralu, G.P., *Ind. J. Pharm, Sci.*, 1982, **44**(1), Suppl. 1-34.
65. Mahashar, K.S., Caius, J.F., *Ind. Med. Res. Memo.*, 1931, **19**, 10.
66. Saha, J.C., Kalyanasundaram, S., *Ind. J. Med. Res.*, 1962, **50**(6), 881.

2
Allium sativum Linn

Garlic, botanically known as *Allium sativum* Linn (Family-Liliaceae) is one of the most commonly used spices. The plant is widely cultivated in India and many other parts of the world.

Garlic occurs as a sub-globular, compound bulb greyish white, 4 to 6 cms in diameter with several (8-20) cloves, the whole surrounded by 3-5 whitish, papery membranous scales from the leaf bases of the previous years bulb and terminating in a thick papery out growth. The cloves are attached to a flattened circular, woody axis with numerous thin, wiry roots on the underside and short, sub-cylindrical out growth on the upper surface.

Each clove is ovoid, 3-4 sided surrounded by two papery scale leaves, the outer one whitish and loose, the inner one pink and adherent, but easily separable from the solid portion of the clove. These papery scale leaves enclose two whitish, fleshy scales, the inner one thinnery and smaller than the outer. Two yellowish brown, conduplicate (right) half of the leaf is folded upon the left half lengthwise foliage leaves present in the centre. Odour, when brushed strongly alliaceous, taste persistently pungent, alliaceous.

Under microscope, cloves show a number of concentric bulblets, each bulblet, 5-10 mm. in diameter, consists of an outer scale, an epidermis, a ground tissue and a layer of lower epidermal cells. Dry scales consist of 2-3 layers of cells rectangular in appearance but with broadly angular slant and walls. These cells contain plenty of rhomboid crystals of calcium oxalate. The upper epidermal cells next to the dry scale layer consist of rectangular to cubical cells of one layer next to which there are several layers of large parenchymatous cells among which there are interspaced many vascular bundles each of which consists of xylem and pholem arranged alternately. Lower epidermis consists of cubical cells which are much smaller than the upper epidermal cells. The same series of arrangement of tissues is met within different bulblets which are arranged in concentric adjustment. 2 to 3 such bulblets are arranged concentrically (Mukerji, 1953).

PHYTOCHEMICAL WORK

Stoll and Seeback (1948) isolated the active principles of garlic in the pure crystalline form. This active principle, named alliin, was found to be (+). 8-allyl- - cystein- sulphoxide with the following chemical formula (Stoll et al, 1951, 1953).

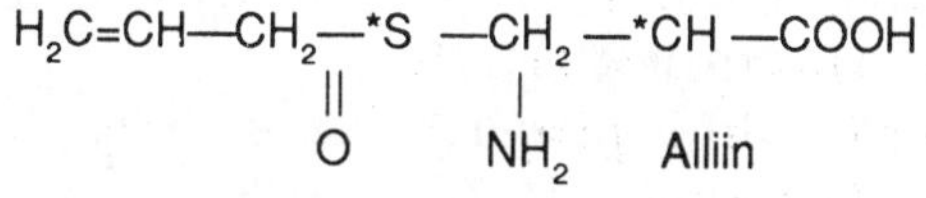

$$H_2C=CH—CH_2—^*S —CH_2 —^*CH —COOH$$
$$\overset{\|}{O} \quad \overset{\|}{NH_2} \quad \text{Alliin}$$

Electronic Formula

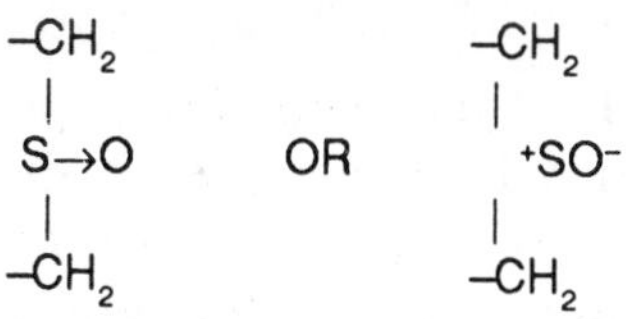

$$\begin{array}{ccc} -CH_2 & & -CH_2 \\ | & & | \\ S{\rightarrow}O & OR & ^+SO^- \\ | & & | \\ -CH_2 & & -CH_2 \end{array}$$

Sulphur and carbon marked with the asterisk in the chemical formula show asymmetric centres in the molecule so theoretically three optical isomers of alliin are possible, which have also been prepared synthetically.

Alliin (a non-bactericidal compound) is a precursor of a highly bactericidal substance, allicin (Cavallito and Bailey, 1944, 1945). Alliin is very rapidly decomposed to allicin, pyruvic acid and ammonia by the highly specific enzyme, alliinase which is present in the garlic, Alliinase is capable of splitting(-)-S-allyl-L- cystein isomer of alliin, the reaction rate being slower but is does not attach either of the D-cystein isomers (Stoll et al, 1948, 1949, 1951). As soon as any part of the plant is damaged the enzyme alliinase gets activated and splits alliin with the formation of allicin which has the characteristic odour of garlic. further decomposition of alliin yields the volatile sharply odourous allyl sulphide.

Besides this, a number of other antibiotic principles have also been isolated, namely, allistatin I, allistatin II (Datta et al, 1948)[8] and garlicin (Watt and Breyer-Brandwijk, 1962)[9].

A brief account of the chemical constituents of garlic based on the information available in the literature is given in Table I.

A review of research work reported on tissue culture studies on garlic revealed that Havranek (1972) was the first person to develop the virus free garlic clones from meristematic culture. Later on Havranek and Novak (1973) introduced garlic into the tissue culture system and reported the bud formation in the callus cultures. The studies on cytogenetics of cultured somatic cells, regeneration ability of long term callus cultures and phenotypic characteristics of the plants regenerated in vitro with their cytological status have been carried out by Novak (1974, 1980, 1981)., Novak and Havranek (1975).

Since garlic is sexually sterile and progagated strictly by cloves and bulbils (Novak and Havranek, 1975) meristem and callus culture is a means by which virus free plants could be produced. In addition to virus free production, genetic variability or restoration of fertility may occur in plants differentiated from callus.

Culture of garlic callus from leaf explants has been developed on Murashige and Skoog's (MS) basal medium supplemented with IAA, 2, 4-D and kinetin. The same basal medium supplemented with IAA and kinetin induced shoot formation. Kehr and Schaefer (1976) obtained callus from 3 mm. garlic apices cultured on MS basal medium containing IAA. kinetin, 2, 4-D and coconut milk. The organogenesis, leading to the formation of shoots was observed when the callus cultures were transferred into the same medium without 2,4-D. In vitro propagation of garlic by shoot proliferation has been reported by Bhojwani and Sant (1980). Organogenesis as well as embryogenesis in callus obtained from garlic stem tip, leaf and stem explants on a chemically defined medium has been reported by El-Nil Abo in 1977. The plantlets and embryoids regenerated from the callus cultures were virus free but filamentous virus particles were noted in callus cultures initiated from stem tips or from bulb leaf explants. The data presented do not provide conclusive evidence, that the regenerated parts are completely free of viruses El-Nill Abo, 1977).

Medicinal Value of Garlic

The medicinal importance of garlic had been recognised by different schools of medicine both indigenous as well as foreign since time immemorial. Some of the important medicinal uses of garlic as enumerated by Kirtikar and Basu (1935) are listed in Table II.

To give a scientific basis for the ancient claims regarding the therapeutic efficacy of garlic in various diseases and disorders, a large number of experiments have been carried out on different experimental models. As a result of these experiments garlic has been found to be of value both in human beings and animals in conditions like-

1) Cancer (Weisberger and Pensky, 1957), Hartwell, 1968).
2) Diabetes (Laland and Haverevold, 1933).
3) Hypertension (Loeper and De Bray, 1921).
4) Arteriosclerosis (Watt and Breyer-Brandwilk, 1962).
5) Angina pectoris (Fortunatov, 1952).
6) Chronic colitis and gastritis (Fortunatov, 1952).
7) Rheumatoid arthritis (Medicinal Plants of India, Vol. I, 1962).
8) Helminthiasis (Rico, 1928, Vinson, 1941).
9) Amoebiasis and other protozoal infections (Watt and Breyer-Brandwijk, 1962)[9].
10) Bacterial and fundal infections (Datta, et al, 1948, Dubrova, 1950, Mukerji, 1953).

Results of these studies justify the multifarious roles, played by garlic in the ancient systems of medicine.

Table 2.1 Chemical Composition of Garlic (Expressed in Gram Per 100 Gram of Except Otherwise Stated)

S.No.	Constitutent	Percentage	Reference
1.	Water	62.20	The Wealth of India, 1948 Bhandari and Mukerji, 1959.
2.	Protein	06.30	-do-
3.	Fat 00.10	-do-	-do-
4.	Carbohydrates	29.00	Ananthkrishnan and Venkatarama, 1941
	A. Reducing sugar	00.14	-do-
	B. Starch	08.22	-do-
	C. Sucrose	03.79	-do-
	D. Dextrin	07.69	-do-
	E. Inulin	Not reported	Braecke, 1921
	F. Sinistrin	-do-	Rundqvist, 1909
5.	Volatile oils	0.10-0.90	Watt and Breyer Brandwijk, 1962
	A. Diallyl-Disulphide	60.00	Semmler, 1892 and 1906
	B. Allyl-Propyl-disulphide	06.00	-do-
	C. Diallyl-trisulphide	Not reported	-do-
	D. Diallyl-polysulphide	-do-	-do-
	E. Diallyl-sulphide		-do-
	F. An unidentified higher boiling fraction	-do-	-do-
6.	Minerals		
	A. Calcium	00.03	The Wealth of India, 1948[29]
	B. Phosphorus	00.31	-do-
	C. Iron	01.30mg	-do-
	D. Zinc	01.00mg (Fresh Bulb)	Bertrand and Benzon, 1928[36];
		00.17mg (Dry bulb)	Idem, 1928[37]
		03.40mg (Ash)	
	E. Iodine	Not reported	Krosber, 1927[38]

S.No. Constitutent	Percentage	Reference
7. Vitamins		
A. Vitamin C	13.00mg	Bhandari and Mukerji, 1959[30]
B. Vitamin A	Not reported	-do-
C. Vitamin B	-do-	-do-
D. Vitamin D	-do-	Parino and Dominici, 1926[39]
8. Enzymes and Hormones		Glaser et. al. 1939[40]
A. Peroxidase	Not reported	Sugihera and Cruese, 1925[41]
B. Catalase	-do-	Watt and Breyer-Brandwijk, 1962[5]
C. Alliinase	-do-	Stoll et. al, 1948[2], 1951[3], 1953[4].
D. Male and female hormones	-do-	Glaser et.al. 1939[40]
9. Nitrogen content		
A. Non-protein nitrogen	67.00	Anantkrishnan and Venkataraman, 1941[31]
B. Protein nitrogen	29.34	Parthasarthi and Sastry, 1959[42]
10. Amino Acids		Greenstein and Winitz, Ed., 1961[43]
A. Essential Amino Acids		-do-
B. Sulphur containing Amino Acids		-do-
i) Methionine	230.00mg (In protein) 177.00mg (Free)	
C. Amino-Acids without sulphur		
i) Lysine	277.00 mg (In protein) 105.00 mg. (Free)	Parthasarathi and Sastry, 1959[42] -do-
ii) Histidine	061.00 mg (In protein) 830.00 mg. (Free)	-do-
iii) Arginine	450.00 mg.	-do-

S.No.	Constitutent	Percentage	Reference
iv)	Threonine	(In protein) 596.00 mg. (Free) 153.00 mg.	-do-
v)	Valine	(In protein) 1001.00 mg. (Free) 243.00 mg.	Parthasarathi and Sastry, 1959.
vi)	Isoleucine	(In protein) 054.00 mg. (Free) 0.93.00 mg	-do-
vii)	Leucine	(In protein) 0.24.00 mg. (Free) 144.00 mg.	-do-
viii)	Phenylalanine	(In protein) 047 00 mg. (Free) 0.86.00 mg.	-do-
B.	Non-essential Amino Acids		
i)	Cystein	(In protein) 029.00 mg (Free) Absent in protein 032.00 mg. (Free)	-do-
ii)	Alliin	800.00 mg. (Free)	Atal and Sethi, 1961

S.No.	Constitutent	Percentage	Reference
b)	Amino Acids without sulphur		
i)	Alanine	137.00 mg (in protein) 066.00 mg (Free)	Parthasarathi and Sastry, 1959.
ii)	Aspartic Acid	236.00 mg. (in protein) 131.00 mg (Free)	-do-
iii)	Glutamic Acid	163.00 mg (in protein) 270.00 mg. (Free)	-do-
iv)	Glycine	109.00 mg (in protein) 096.00 mg (Free)	
v)	Proline	118.00 mg (in protein) 105.00 mg (Free)	-do-
vi)	Serine	118.00 mg (In protein) 083.00 mg (Free)	-do-
vii)	Tyrosine	147.00 mg (in protein) 080.00 mg (Free)	Parthasarathi and Sastry, 1959
viii)	Tryptophan	061.00 mg	-do-

S.No.	Constitutent	Percentage	Reference
11. Miscellaneous			
A.	Tuberoholoside	(in protein) 120.00 mg (Free) 10.00	Watt and Breyer-Brandwijk. 1962[9]
B.	A sulphur containing glucoside	Not reported	Braecke, 1921.
C.	Saponin	-do-	Koczwara, 1949[43]
D.	An ether-soluble, steam Volatile alkaloidal substance	-do-	Laland & Havreveld, 1933.
E.	An alkaloidal product (m.p.174oC)	-do-	-do-
F.	Hydrocyanic Acid	Not reported	Quisumbing, 1947
G.	Phytonoides	-do-	Tokin, 1946.
H.	Allyl-2-propane 1-thiosulphinate	-do-	Watt and Breyer-Brandwijk, 1962
I.	Allyl-thiosulphinates	-do-	-do-

Table 2.2 Medicinal Uses of Garlic in Indigenous System of Medicine

S.No.	Dis-order of-	Uses
1.	Gastro-intestinal tract	Carminative, antiflatulent, appetiser, gastric stimulant, digestive, in atonic dyspepsin, duodenal ulcer, gastro intestinal catarrh, piles and others.
2.	Respiratory tract	Expectorant in bronchitis, bronchial asthma, pulmonary phthisis, pulmonary tuberculosis, laryngeal tuberculosis, gangrene of lung, whooping cough.
3.	Miscellaneous type	Rubefacient, counterirritant, anti-septic, tonic, anti-convulsant, analgesic, anti-pyretic, anti-inflammatory, anti-rheumatic, anti-tumor, diuretic, emmenagogue aphrodisiac, in cardio-vascular diseases.

References

1. Mukerji, B., in "Indian Pharmaceutical Codex I' 1953, New Delhi: CSIR India.
2. Stoll, A. & Seebeck, E., Sci. Indust. Res. 7(1). 45, 1948.
2. Atal, C.K. & Sethi, J.K. Curr. Sci. 30(9), 338, 1961.
3. Stoll, A. and Seebeck, E., in 'Advances in Enzymology', (Intersciences Publishers, Inc, New York), 11, 377, 1951.
4. Stoll, A., The Indian Pharmacist, 8(8), 349, 1953.
5. Cavallito, C.Y. & Bailey, J.H. J. Amer. Chem. Soc., 66, 1950, 1944.
6. Cavallito, C.J., Bailey, J.H. & Buck, J.S. J. Amer. Chem. Soc., 67, 1032, 1945.
7. Stoll. A. and Seebeck, E., Helv. Chim. Acta. 32, 866, 1949.
8. Datta. N.L. Krishnamurthi, A & Siddiqui, S., J. Sci. Industr. Res. 7(B), 42, 1948.
9. Watt, J.M. Breyer-Brandwijk, M.G., 'The Medicinal and Poisonous Plants of Southern and Eastern Africa. (Ed. II), pp. 674, 1962.   (E & S. Livingstone Ltd. Edinburgh and London).
10. Havranek, P., Ochrana rostlin (Praha), 8, 291, 1972 (in Czech.)
11. Havranek, P. & Novak, F.J., Z. Pflanzenphysiol., 68, 308, 1973.
12. Novak, F.J., Caryologia, 27, 45, 1974.
13. Novak, F.J., Z. Pflanzenzuchtg. 85, 250, 1980
14. Novak, F.J., Cytologia (Tokyo), 46, 371, 1981.
15. Hartwell, J.L., Lloydia, 31, 72, 1968.
15. Novak, F.J., & Havranek, P., Acta, Fac. Rer. Natur., Univ. Comenianze. Genetica (Bratislava), 5, 143, 1975.
16. Kehr, A.E. & Schaeffer, G.W., Hort, Science, 11(4), 422, 1976.
17. Bhojwani A., Sant. S., Sci. Hortic, 13(i), 47, 1980.
18. El-Nil, Abo, Plant Sci. Lett., 9(3), 259, 1977.
19. Kirtikar, K.R. & Basu, B.D., in "Indian Medicinal Plants', (Ed. 2nd Vol.4) pp. 2513, 1935.
20. Weisberger, A.S. & Pansky, J., Science, 126, 1112, 1957.
22. Konoshima & Yamamota, 1970, in Pharm. J., 206., 341, 1971.

22. Laland, P. & Havrevold, Hoppe-Seyl. Z., 221, 180, 1933.
23. Loeper & Debray, Bull, Soc. Med., 37, 1032, 1921.
24. Fortunatov, M.M., C.A., 46, 8811, 1952.
25. 'Medicinal Plants of India'. Vol. I, Indian Council of Medical Research, New Delhi, pp. 40. 1962.
26. Rico, T.J., Compt. Rend. Soc. Biol, 95, 1997, 1926, C.A., 22, 464, 1928.
27. Vinson, L. Rev. Agric. Congo, Belge, 22, 208(1941.)
28. Dubrova, G.B. Micrology, Moscow, 19, 229, 1950.
29. The Wealth of Indian Vol. I, pp. 58, 1948 (C.S.I.R., New Delhi).
30. Bhandari, P.R. & Mukerjee, B., Nagarjun 3, 121, 1959.
31. Anant Krishnan, C.P. & Venkataraman, P.R., Proc, Ind. Acad. Sci., 13(B), 129, 1941, C.A. 35, 5160, 1941.
32. Braecke, H., Acad. Roy. Belge. Classe, Sci. Meru., (2) 6 No. 6, 1. 1921, C.A. 17, 2128, 1923.
33. Rundqvist, C. Pharmaceutiskt Notisblad, 18, 323, 1909.
34. Semmler, F.W., Arch Pharm., 230, 434, 1892.
35. Semmler, F.W., Apothekerztg., Berl., 21, 987, 1906.
36. Bertrand, G. & Benzon, B., Bull. Soc. Hyg. Aliment., 16, 457, 1928.
37. Idem, Compt. Rend. 187, 1008, 1020, C.A. 23, 1090, 1929.
38. Krosber, L. Suddeut. Apoth. Ztg., 67, 668, 1927.
39. Parrino, G. & Dominici, A., Annali d' Igiene, 37, 1, 1926.
40. Glaser, E. & Brobrik, R., Arch. Exptl. Path. Pharmakol 193, 1, 1939, C.A., 34, 3283, 1940.
41. Sugihera, J. and Cruess, W.V. J., Fruit Products, J., 24, 297, 1925, C.A., 40, 6508, 1940.
42. Parthasarathi, K. & Sastry, C.A., Indian J. Pharmacy, 21, 283, 1959.
43. Greenstein, J.P. & Winitz Milton, in Chemistry of the Amino Acid's, (Vo., 1, Ed. 1961). pp. 2662.
43. Koczwara, M., Publ. Pharm. Comm. Pol. Acad. Sci., 1, 65, 1949. C.A. 46, 10548, 1952.
44. Quisumbing, E., Phillipp. J. For., 5, 145, 1947.
45. Telle, J. and Gautheret, R., Compt., Rend. 224, 1653, 1947.
45. Tokin, B. Am. Rev. Soviet Med., 1, 237, 1944.

3
Cassia alata Linn

Cassia alata Linn. is known by different vernacular names in different regions which are as follows — English: Ring worm shrubs; Hindi: Dad murdun; Telugu : Metta-Tamara; Marathi: Dadoo Murdun; Tamil: Wandukall Seemee-Aghatie; Sinhalese: Attora; Burmese: Maizaligi; Sanskrit: Dad-rughna.

Cassia alata Linn. is Dicotyledonous gymnosperm, it belongs to Archichlamydeae group in which it belongs to the order: Rosales

Suborder	:	Leguminosineae
Family	:	Leguminosae
Subfamily	:	Caesalpinaedae
Genera	:	Cassia, having anthracene derivatives.

Cassia alata Linn. (Fig. 3.1) is a large shrub 8-12 ft in height; with very thick finely downy but spreading, irrgularly angled, glabrous branches. Leaves are subsile, 5-15 cm long, 8-12 in pairs, oblong-obtuse; minutely mucronate, rigidly subcoriaceous, glabrous or obscurely downy beneath, broadly rounded, oblique at the base. Rhachis narrowly winged on each side of the face, stipules deltoid, rigid, persistent, articulate, 6mm long. Flowers in short pedicles, in spiciform pedunculate racemes, the buds in yellow caducous bracts. Sepals obtuse; petals bright yellow with darker veins, broad ovate 3-4 cm long. Stamens very unequal, perfect stamen 7. The anthers are subequal or those of 2-3 lowest larger than others, 3 posterior filaments without anthers. Pods long, lingulate with a broad wing down the middle of each valve, membranous, dehiscent straight and glabrous 10-12 cm long and 1.3-1.6 cm broad. Seeds 30 or more in each pod.

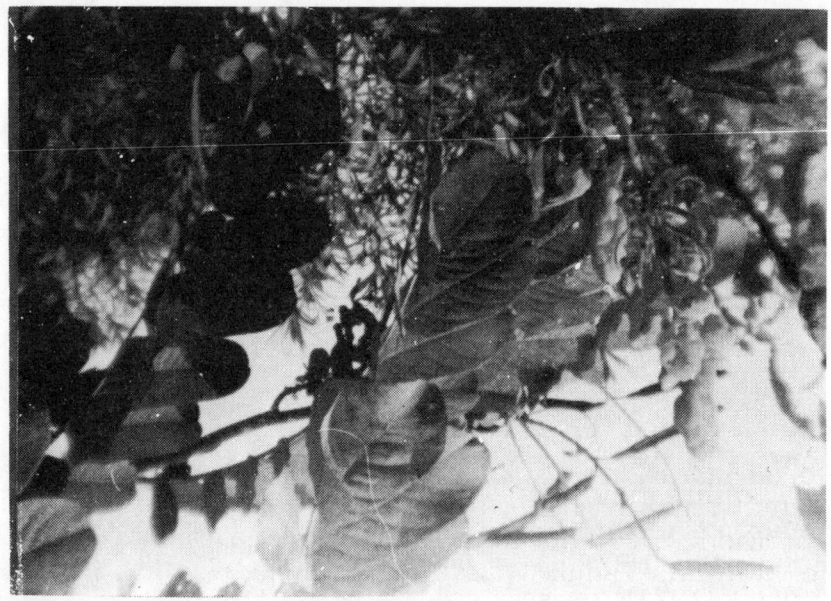

Fig. 3.1 *Cassia alata* Linn

Cassia alata Linn, is native of the West Indies and was introduced into India, cultivated mainly in Travancore.

The following phytochemical work has already been reported on *Cassia alata* Linn...

Hauptmann et-al (1950)[1] reported rhein (1.8 dihydroxy anthraquinone-3 carboxylic acid); glucose and Rhamnose as sugar moiety. A yellow dibasic acid $C_{15}H_8O_7$ (melting point 335-336°) and some unidentified anthraquinone derivatives also reported. The results indicate the relation of this species to the Cassia species of senna leaves.

Anchel (1950)[2] confirmed the presence of yellow crystalline dibasic acid $C_{15}H_8O_7$ (melting point 335-336°C) obtained by Hauptmann et al, while working on Cassia reticulata along Cassia alata Linn..

Toledo (1950)[3] studied the pharmacognosy of *Cassia alata* Linn. and tested the anthraquinone derivatives with Borntrager-Wasicky reaction.

R. Tiwari and B.K. Singh (1943)[4] further isolated β-sitosterol, chrysophanol and some fatty acids and seed fats from the Cassia alata Linn.

Tiwari (1953)[5], reported three colouring matter in the seeds. A yellow compound (melting point 194°), soluble in alkali, $C_{15}H_{10}O_4$ identical with chrysophanic acid, another yellow substance $C_{13}H_8O_4$ (melting point 187°) soluble in alkali and a red coloured compound $C_{11}H_8O_4$ having melting point 212°. Besides these three, two other colouring matters were also isolated, namely 2 methyl anthraquinone and Protocatechuic acid.

Tiwari and Yadav (1971)[6] reported that the seed of the *Cassia alata* Linn. contain some hydroxy anthraquinone; chrysophanol and β-sitosterol (Tiwari 1965)[7] and some fatty acid and seed fat (Tiwari 1941)[8]. He reported two new anthraquinone moieties in the root of the Cassia alata Linn. and also confirmed their structures using I.R. UV spectra and chemical degradation studies. The two new anthraquinones are: 1,3,8 trihydroxy-2 methyl anthraquinone (melting point 232°) and 1,5 dihydroxy-8-methoxy-2 methyl anthraquinone-3-0-β-D (+)-glucopyranoside (melting point 180°).

Mopett (1971)[9] revised the structure for cassiollin. Cassiollin is 1,7 dihydroxy-8-methoxycarbonyl 3-methyl xanthone i.e. pinselin and not 1,7 dihydroxy 5 methoxy carbonyl 3-methyl xanthose as previously reported.

Rao et al (1975)[10], first time reported the presence of Aloe-emodin and 217-sitosterol using chromotography over alumina using leaves extract. The results were further confirmed by using Thin Layer Chromatography.

Rai (1978)[11] has reported the latest work on the leaves and pods of Cassia alata Linn. of Indian origin. He reported that reduced anthraquinone compounds are present in leaves and quinone pigments in the roots of Cassia alata Linn... He further reported the roughly quantity of the anthraquinones present in the leaves and pods hence showed fruit (pod) contain more anthraquinones than leaves.

Smith and Ali (1979)[12] worked on the leaves of Cassia alata Linn. of Fiji variety and also summarise the constituents of the leaves by previous workers. He reported, the first study Hauptmann and Nazaria (1950) led the isolation of the rhein, glucose and cassiaxanthone (Nair et al 1970)[13]. Kaempferol, rhein, aloe-emodin by Rai (1978)[11]. In three recent studies, chromatography has been used to identify chrysophanol, emodin, rhein and aloe-emodin (Vallaroya and Barnel-Santos 1976)[14], aloe-emoduin and glycoside of rhein and aloe-emodin (Rai, 1978), chrysophanol, aloe-emodin and anthraquinone glycosides (Harrison and Virginia 1977)[15].

Contradictory to above, Smith and Ali (1979)[12] reported iso-chrysophanol instead of chrysophanol which is a isomer differing only in melting point and physcion-1-glucose present in the Cassia alata Linn. leaves of Fiji variety.

Gupta et al (1980)[16] showed the presence of tertiary alkaloid (including primary and secondary) in the leaves, stems and flowers part of *Cassia alata* Linn. He only performed the test for alkaloid.

Benjamin (1980)[17] isolated and analysed the volatile constituents present in the *Cassia alata* Linn. The volatile oil fraction consisted of Sesquiterpenes and some phenolic compounds.

The following uses and pharmacological work has already been reported on the *Cassia alata* Linn.

Cassia alata Linn. is reputed for its medicinal values in Ayurveda, The leaves are sour; cure "vata" itching, cough, asthma, ring worm, skin diseases, vermicide (Kirtikar and Basu, 1933)[18].

Kirtikar and Basu (1933)[18] reported many uses of Cassia alata Linn. In snake bite the fresh leaves are given internally. For scropion's sting any part of the plant is made into paste and applied to the sting. The leaves of Cassia alata Linn. are regarded as an excellent medicine for ring worm. They are also used in other skin diseases. According to them leaves of the plant as paste with lime juices, externally applied is excellent cure of ring worm. This fact is further supported by Fox (1952)[19] who reported its use as antiherpetic in Phillipines. The leaves have also purgative properties. In their investigations, Kirtikar and Basu obtained best results by washing the part affected by eczema, repeatedly with strong decoction of leaves and flowers. Bark has same property. According to them the leaves and flowers prescribed internally as a tonic. They further reported that in case of asthma and bronchitis, in herpetic constitution, the decoction of leaves and flowers should be taken in repeated doses during the day, relieving dyspnoeal appression and promoting expectoration.

Koman (1920)[20] in his investigation reported that leaves are effective against ring worm, and skin diseases as mentioned by

Kartikar and Basu. But in chronic cases the drug failed to bring about a cure.

According to Kirtikar and Basu the drug acts on the bowel slightly and increase the secretion of urine, i.e. acts as a diuretic. This fact supported the use of roots of Cassia alata Linn. as a diuretic in West Indies.

Kirtikar and Basu (1933)[18] further reported that in the different region, the leaves of *Cassia alata* Linn, are used in a different way against skin affection. In Guinea, the pounded fresh leaves are rubbed on the affected part. In Gold Coast, the leaves are crushed and mixed with black pepper and applied to dhoby itch, craw-craw and ring worm on the head or on the skin. The infected place is rubbed until the blood comes and then the leaves are rubbed in the palm and applied to the sores, which are effectively cured. This is one of the most effective amongst native medicine, When boiled the leaves have a purgative effect. They are also boiled and consumed by women to hasten the delivery of children.

Mhaskas and Cains (1933)[21] contradicted Kirtikar and Basu, in that the leaves are not antidote to snakevenom. Every part of the plant is equally useless in the treatment of scorpion sting.

Mariam (1947)[22] showed the antibiotic effect of *Cassia alata* Linn. leaves against Staphyllococcus aureus and Escherichia coli using Oxford cup method. She showed that alcoholic extract is effective but water extract is ineffective as antibiotic.

Isuine (1947)[23] reported the insecticidal value of the Cassia alata Linn. shrub, and said chrysophanic acid present in the plant responsible for insecticidal activity of the shrub. He also reported the use of Cassia alata Linn. as insecticide and against skin disease among the West Africans.

Scharpenseel et al (1948)[24] has also confirmed the anti-bacterial property of Cassia alata Linn..

Fox (1952)[19] further supported the use of juices of the leaves of *Cassia alata* Linn. as antiherpetic and skin diseases in Phillipines.

Bungi and Plana (1960)[25], observed the fungistatic action of the leaves in alcoholic extract, against some mycotic organisms e.g. T. mentogrophytes, M. gypseum, E. floccosum, etc. In other words they further confirmed the use of Cassia alata Linn.

against skin diseases and reported that chrysophanic acid was responsible for it.

Montelleno (1975)[26] showed that cathartic action of the drug is due to the presence of chrysophanic acid and its glycosides. The reduction product of chrysophanol i.e. chrysorbin is used topically for psoriasis and other chronic skin diseases.

Radhakrishnan et al (1976)[27] observed the antifungal activity of various extracts against various micro-organisms e.g. T. ajeloi, T. mentagraphite, M. gypseum, M. cookei, etc. The result showed the antifungal activity observed only in organic extracts e,g. extract of petroleum ether, acetone, chloroform, etc. but not in aqueous extracts. He also prescribed the decoction of leaves taken internally for skin affection and as a blood purifier in germ infestation.

Holdsworth (1980)[28] confirmed the antibiotic action of leaves. He also studied the drug against eczema and reported the use of drug in Queensland (Australia) against eczema.

Benjamin et al (1981)[17] isolated the volatile fraction consist of sesquiterpenes and phenolic compounds. He studied the antimicrobial activity of the drug against gram positive and gram negative bacteria including pseudomonas and reported that volatile fraction is responsible for this activity.

Deb (1981)[29] mentioned the economic significance of Cassia alata Linn. alongwith its uses. Abraham et al (1981)[30] mentioned the Cassia alata Linn. among the medicinal plant used in Israel. Morrison et al (1982)[31] showed the effect of *Cassia alata* Linn. on blood sugar level in the dog. Sadique (1982)[32] showed the biochemical mode of action of some herbal medicines including *Cassia alata*. Smith et al (1983)[33] confirmed the use of *Cassia alata* Linn. as pesticide in agriculture.

Bhat (1985)[34] confirmed the two possible uses of Cassia alata Linn.. First in the treatment of constipation in which he prescribed the powder of sun dried leaves alongwith potassium aluminium sulphate taken orally two teaspoon full at the time of need. Second in the treatment of ring-worm.

The above mentioned uses denote the importance of Cassia alata Linn. in the medicine. The name ringworm shrub itself shows the effectiveness of drug against skin diseases besides cathartic, purgative action. Blood purifier, insecticidal activity, antibiotic activity and fungistatic action further enhance its importance. If taken orally it is used to relieve the constipation, bronchitis and asthma.

Shah et al (1968)[35] reported that the efficacy of Cassia species (in general) in skin diseases might be attributed to anthraquinone derivatives especially to chrysophanol.

The literature survey both phytochemical as well as pharmacological showed that Cassia alata Linn. is considered as an important medicinal plant not only in India but in other countries as well. It had been of immense interest for many research workers, in different parts of world including Indian subcontinent, with different organic parts of different time period, and with different mode of research procedures and manipulations. A wide variety of therapeutic findings have been reported using different plant parts e.g. root shows diuretic action. The findings ofcourse are not due to one and the same class of compounds, namely anthraquinone derivatives, due to which the plant seems to have its importance as a medicine, as a purgative and in skin diseases.

References

1. Hauptmann. H, et al. "Some constituents of the leaves of Cassia alata." Jour. of American Chemical Society, **72**, 1492-1495, 1950.
2. Anchel, M. " Identity of a substance isolated from Cassia reticulata with that isolated from Cassia alata." Jour. of American Chemical Society, 72, 1832, 1950.
3. Toledo, A.N. "Pharmacognostic study of Cassia alata". Anais faculdade farm.e.odontal Univ. Sao Paulo, Brazil 7, 105-113, 1950.
4. Tiwari, R., Singh, B.K. "Chemical examination of Cassia alata Linn. Part-I. The component acids of the fatty oil from seeds.. Proc. Natural Academic Sciences-India, 13A (2), 141, 1943.
5. Tiwari, R. (1953). "Chemical examination of seeds of *Cassia alata*-isolation of colouring matter". Proc. 40th Indian Science Congress-Pt (III), 349, 1953.
6. Tiwari, R.B. and Yadav, O.P. "Structural study of the quinone pigments from the root of Cassia alata". Planta Medica, 19 (4), 296, 1971.

7. Tiwari, R.B., Planta Medica, 24 (6), 149, 1965.

8. Tiwari R.B.J. Sci. Ind. Res. 8C, 245-248, 1941.

9. Mopett, C.E. "Revised Structure for Cassialin; Identity with Pinselin". Chemical Communication 9 D, 423-424, 1971.

10. Rao, J.V. et al. "Occurrence of kaempferol and aloe emodin in the leaves of Cassia alata Linn." Current Science, 44 (20), 736-737, 1975.

11. Rai, P.P, "Anthracene derivatives in leaves and fruits of Cassia alata". Current Science 47 (8), 271-272, 1978.

12. Smith and Ali. "Anthraquinones from the leaves of Cassia alata from Fiji." New Zealand Journal of Science, 22 (2), 123-125, 1979.

13. Nair et al. Phytochem., 12 (3), 392, 1970.

14. Vallaroya et al. Phytochem., 6 (2), 514, 1976.

15. Harrison et al. J. Crude Drug Research, 18 (1), 33-44, 1977.

16. Gupta, M.P. et al. "Alkaloid Screening of Panamanian plants". Quarterly Journal of Crude Drug Research 18(3), 105-125, 1980.

17. Benjamin, T.V. et al. "Investigation of Cassia alata, plant used in Nigeria in the treatment of skin-diseases". Quarterly Jour. of Crude drug Research 19. (2 and 3), 93-96, 1981.

18. Kirlikar and Basu *Indian Medicinal Plants"* vol. II, 2nd Ed 1933. p. 856, 870.

19. Fox, R.B. "The Pintube Negritos, their useful plants and material plants of American origin". Philipines Jour. of Science, 81 (324), 173-213, 1952.

20. Koman, M.C. "Report on the investigation of Indiginous drugs." 3rd Report. 1920, pp. 20.

21. Mhaskas and Cains. "Indian plant remedies used in snake-bite". Indian Medical Research, Memo No. 19 and 28, 1931.

22. Mariam. M., George, J. Sci. Industrial Research, 6B (3), 42-48, 1947.

23. Isuine, F.R. "West African Insecticide", Colonial Plant Animal products, 5 (1), 34-38, 1947.

24. Scharpenseel *et al* "Prelimenary studies on Antibacterial principal in flowering plants" Araneta J. Agricullure, 3 (2), 46-55 1948.

25. Bungi, E and Plana. "The antifungal activity of Cassia alata". Manila, Cento Escalar University, p-160. Phillipines abstracts, 1 (3), 165, 1960.

26. Montalleno, B.O.de. "Empirical Aztec medicine". Science, 188, Iss. no 4185, 215-220, 1975.

27. Radhakrishnan et al. "Antifungal activity of medicinal plants". Jour. of Research of Ind. Med. Yoga and Homoeopathy 11 (2), 70-73, 1976.

28. Holdsworth, D.K. "Traditional medicinal plants of Northern Solomans. Province Papua Guinea." Quarterly Jour. of Crude drug Research, 18 (1), 33-44, 1980.

29. Deb, D.B., *Economic plants of Tripura state"*, Ind Forests. 107(p), 578-582, 1981.

30. Abraham *et al* "Potentialities of the Isrel flora for medicinal purpose". Fitotrapia *52* (5), 195-200, 1981.

31. Morrison *et al* "Preliminary study of the effects of some West Indies medicinal plants on the blood sugar levels in the dog" West Indies Medicinal Plants Journal, 31(4), 194, 197, 1976.

32. Sadique *et al* "Biochemical mode of actio of some herbal modicine." Abstraet or the paper presented at International work shop on phamcological and biochamical approaches to medicinal plant held at school of Biological Sciences-Kamaraj Uni, Madurai, 12-15, Oil 1982.

33. Smith, A.E. and Secoy. "Use of floral plants in control of agricultural and domestic posts." Economics and Botany *37*(1). 28-57, 1983.

34. Bhat, R.B., "Some medicinal plants of Nigeria" Jour. Econ. Texon. Botany, 6(1), 161-165, 1985.

35. Shah, C.S., Qadry, S.M.J.S. and Tripathi, M.P., "Indian Cassia species II. Ind J. Pharm., *30*, 282, 1968.

4

Cassia angustifolia Vahl

The earliest mention of senna occurs in the 9th century when it first appeared among the medicaments used by the Arabs and somewhat later among those of the Greeks. It seems that Serapion the elder was the first to describe and recommend senna. Some time afterwards, it was also mentioned as a medicinal plant by an Egyptian Doctor named Isac Judabus.

Although varieties of *Cassia* were recognised in folk medicine many centuries ago as medicinal plants, they were at first employed for other purposes than those customary at the present day. It was not until several centuries later that the true importance of senna as a purgative was recognized. Paracelsus and later Lonicerus, Bock as well as Matthiolus recommended the drug as the most reliable and least harmful of all laexative agents.

About 1850, a number of chemists began investigating the nature of the active principles of senna. The most important finding resulting from the chemical investigations carried out during the 2nd half of the 19th century was that the active principles of senna were derived from anthraquinone and were probably glycosides, though it was not possible to isolate a homogenous crystalline substances. Although it was known that cathartic acid prepared by Dragendorff and Kubly, undoubtedly played an important part. Tschirch and Hiepe were able to demonstrate that the various cathartic acid preparations at that time commercially available were not homogenous compounds but amorphous mixtures of variable composition. The last two investigations subsequently devoted themselves

for a study of the active principles of senna but later workers
e.g. Tutin were unable to confirm their results. Although Tutin
succeeded in isolating a large number of substances from senna,
practically none of these possessed the specific action of the
drug.

In the following decades, research workers once more turned
their attention to other anthroquinone drugs. It was found that
many substances previously regarded as anthraquinone
glycosides exist in the plant in the form of anthranol glycosides,
but is was not until about 1930 that this knowledge, also led to
fruitful results in the investigations on senna which had recently
been resumed.

Straub and Gebhardt (1936)[1] demonstrated that the active
principles of senna must also be glycosides of anthranol. A few
years later, two main active principles of senna in pure crystalline
form were isolated by Stoll and Becker. These two closely related
compounds were designated as Sennoside A and Sennoside B.

The sennosides A and B, the two main genuine active
principles of senna, belong to the anthraquinone glycosides.
They can therefore be split into an aglycone and a sugar. The
sugar component consists of D-glucose while the two aglycone
fractions, termed sennidin A and sennidin B, both derived from
the same anthrone. The parent substance anthraquinone, was
prepared by Laurent as long ago as 1840, by oxidation of
anthracene with nitric acid. Reduction of anthraquinone with
tin and glacial acetic acid yielded anthrone which was
desmotropic with anthranol.

Rhein was ioslated from rhubarb and is the parent substance
of the sennidins. it possesses two hydroxyl groups, viz. one at
position 1 and one at position 8, while the carboxyl group
responsible for its acid character is located in C_3 Alizarin is the
most important of the other hydroxy anthraquinones. It occurs
in madder root in the form of ruberythric acid, a glycoside in
which it is combined with the disaccharide primverose {6 -(b-D-
xyloside) - D - glucose}. The primverose is attached to the
hydroxyl group at position 2 and can be split off relatively
easily with the formation of alizarin. Alizarin is a typical mordant
dye.

Karmic acid is of particular interest because it is of animal
origin, being obtained from the dried bodies of the kermes

insect, the female of a particular variety of cochineal or scale insect. The structural formula of karmic acid is still not quiet certain, and it may be that the hydroxyl group at C_2 and the acetyl group at C_3 should be interchanged.

The structure IV shows two anthrone residuas linked together by a carbon - carbon bridge. It is 10 : 10' - bianthronyl which is prepared synthetically by the union of two molecules of anthrone with elimination of an atom of hydrogen from position 10. The bianthronyl is also the parent substance sennosides A & B.

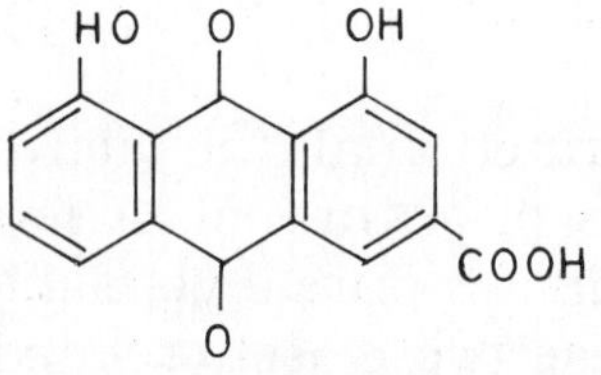

I. Rhein

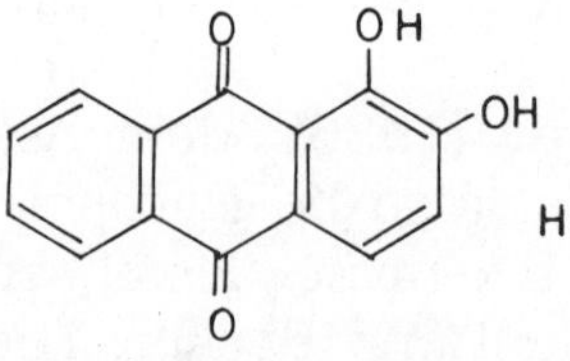

II. Alizarin

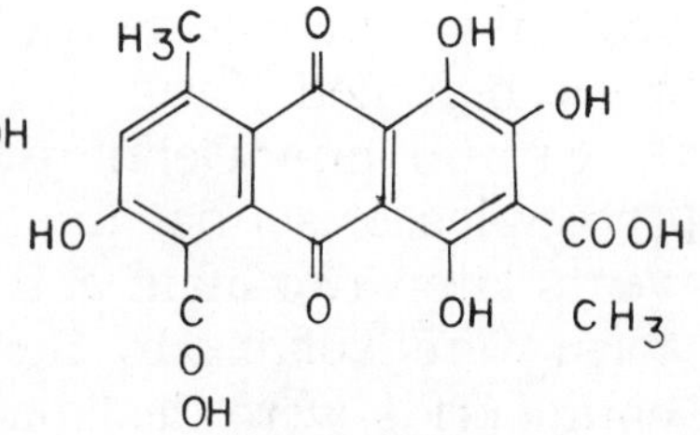

III. Kermic acid

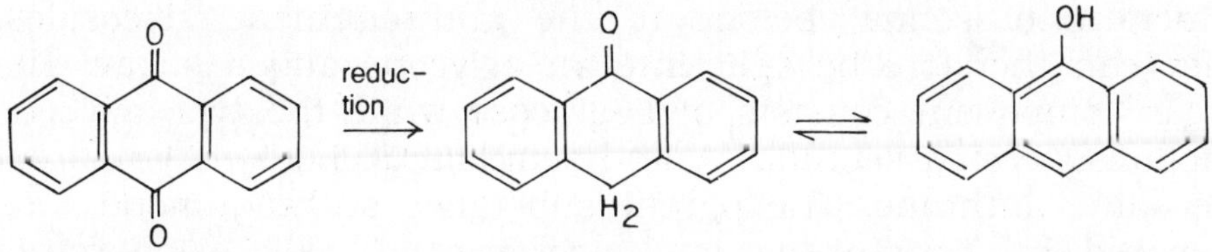

Anthraquinone — reduction → Anthrone ⇌ Anthranol

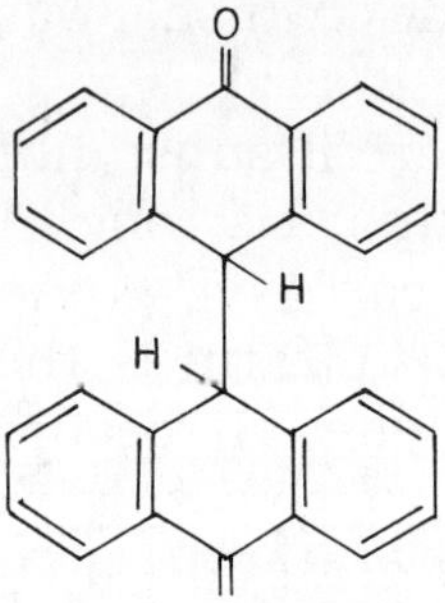

IV. 10:10' Bianthronyl

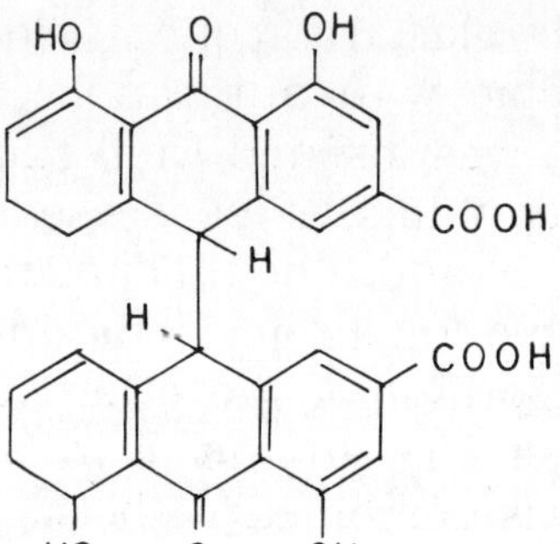

V. Sennidin A & B

The senna aglycones gives a brilliant yellow solution in alkali, the well known red colouration developing only after oxidation. The latter can be effected in various ways. e.g. by exposing to the quartz lamp or by shaking the warm solution with oxygen or air. The nature of the oxidizing agent is, however, important in that it affects the intensity and the shade of the coloration produced. It has been observed that using 3% H_2O_2 as oxidizing agent, an oxidation process can be developed which could be conveniently standardized. This gave a brilliant wine red colour of reproducible intensity. Using this colorimetry a reliable method for the determination of the active glycoside content and senna was secured.

It has been found that the senna glucosides are acids. Owing to the acid nature of these active principles, they are mostly present in the drug as water soluble salts and, in this form, are only extracted in small quantities by anhydrous solvents such as absolute ethanol. Extraction with water results in a very pronounced swelling of the material. Moreover water would also extract enormous quantities of other water soluble compounds present in the drug. The only possible means of extraction therefore is with aquesus organic solvents. Either the glucosides can be converted by means of organic bases into salts which are soluble in organic solvents or else they may be liberated by means of acids and extracted in the form of free acids.

Although the two glycosides sennoside A and sennoside B resemble each other very closely, an exact comparison reveals unmistakable difference in their melting points, solubilities and behavicur during crystallization.

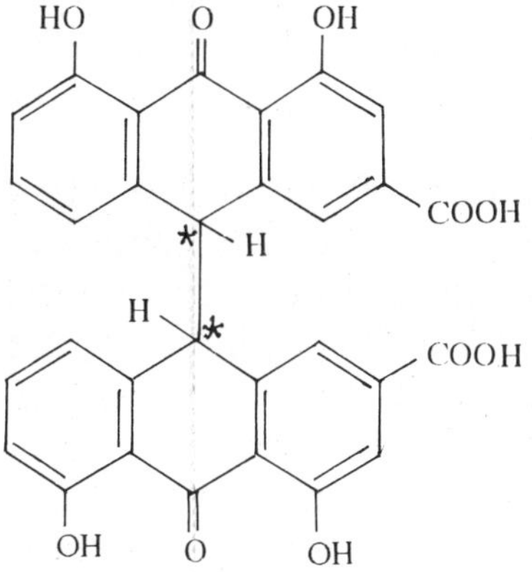

Sennidins A & B

The above formula shows that the sennidin posses two asymetric carbon atoms, one at position 10 and another at position 10'; they are therefore composed of two structurally identical asymmetric systems. Theoretically, four isomers are possible, a (+) form and a (-) form, a racemate and a meso form.

An examination of the sennidins and their derivatives in polarized light has revealed that sennidin A and its derivatives exhibit a strong positive rotation, whereas sennidin b and the compounds derived from it are optically inactive.

A number of compounds have been isolated from drugs, which were presumed to have a 10-10' bianthronyl structure but none of them had shown optical activity. In the above case, rotation of polarized light was first detected on an amorphous preparation of sennidin A. On repeated recrystallization from organic solvents, however the optical rotation decreased rapidly until finally an optically inactive preparation was obtained. Since all samples described in the literature were crystalline, the possibility cannot be excluded that they had lost their optical activity during the very process of recrystallization.

If all these facts be taken into consideration, the difference between sennidin A and sennidin B can be of a purely stereochemical nature. Sennidin A must be the optically active, levorotatory form and ocnnidin B the intramolecularly compensated meso form. If sennidin B were not the meso form but the recemate its glucoside, viz. sennoside B (being a compound of a racemate with D-glucose) would have to be resolvable into D-glucosido - (+) - sennidin i.e. sennoside A. Under all conditions tried so far, sennoside b has behaved as a homogenous compound.

The above formulation of the isomerism between sennoside A and sennoside B is, moreover, in complete harmony with the disappearance of the optical activity on reductive cleavage of sennidin A, as well as with the fact that the monomolecular cleavage products obtained from sennoside A and sennoside B are identical. This identity depends on this fact that, with the disappearance of the asymmetric centre at C_{10}, only the optical activity resulting from the presence of sugar remains.

As far known, it is for the first time that an optically active aglycone of an anthra-glycoside was found among this pharmaceutically and medicinally important class of compounds. Very probably sennidin A is not an isolated instance but represents the prototype of optically active compounds having the dihydro dianthrone structure.

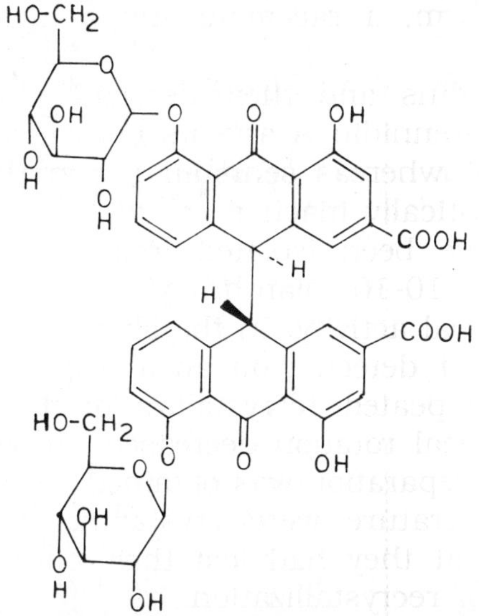

Sennoside A

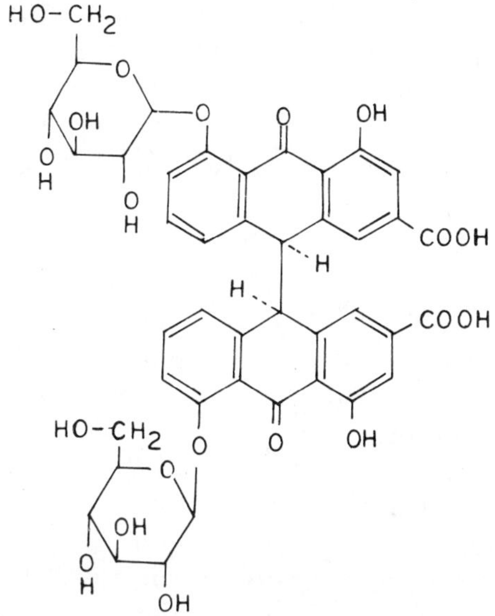

Sennoside B

A list of Cassia species which are known for the anthraquinone content is given below (Chopra *et al.*, 1956)[2] :

1. *C. absus* Linn.
2. *C. angustifolia* Vahl.
3. *C. alata* Linn.
4. *C. auriculata* Linn.
5. *C. burmanni* Wight
6. *C. fistula* Linn
7. *C. glauca* Linn.
8. *C. javanica* Linn
9. *C. mimosoides* Linn.
10. *C. obovata* (L.) Collad.
11. *C. obtusifolia* Linn.
12. *C. occidentalis* Linn.
13. *C. pumila* Lam.
14. *C. siamea* Lam.
15. *C. sophera* Linn.
16. *C. tora* Linn.

C. *angustifolia* Vahl. is known in Hindi as Hindisana; Marathi-Sonamukhi; Bengali-Sanna makki; Tamil-Nilavirai; Telugu-Nela-tangedu; and in Malayalam-Nilavaka.

It is cultivated in South India, Tinnevelly, and Trichinopoly districts. It has been recently introduced in Mysore. The plant is a shrub or undershrub, with pale *subterete or* obtusely angled erect or ascending branches, leaves usually 5-8 jugate, leaflets oval-lanceolate, glabrous; racemes axillary, erect, many flowered, usually considerably exceeding the subtending leaf; Bracts membraneous, ovate or obovate, caducous; Sepals obtuse, membraneous; legume flat, 15-17 mm. in breadth; Seeds obovate, cuneate, compressed, cotyledons plane.

Chemically the leaflets contain Glucosides, Kampferol, anthraquinone, essential oil, isorhamnetin, calcium -oxalate 12% in leaves.

The leaves contains calcium salts, 0.1% of flavanols, isorhamnetin, kaempferol, rhein 0.03% and small amount of emodin.

Khorana and Sanghavi (1964)[3] have done fractioned choromatographic studies and have shown that the pods of C. *angustifolia* contain besides sennoside A and B, glycosides of rhein and chrysophanic acid. Chrysophanic acid was best isolated by acidification of the aqueous extract to pH 3. Biologically, a mixture of these anthraquinone glycoside was more active than either individually. The possibility of the presence of traces of aloe-emodin or emodin glucoside was also indicated.

Dane *et. al.* (1972)[4] studied the development of free and combined anthraquinone in c. *angustifolia* during growth. Colorimetric method was employed and it showed the formation of free anthraquinones in 72 hours and formation of glycosides in a week old seedling.

Chakravarti *et al.* (1955, 1956)[5,6] examined the seeds of C. *angustifolia, C. auriculata, C. fistula, C. laevigata, C. siamea, C. spohera* and C. *tora* and their sterol content. The sterol from C. *siamea* has been identified as α-sitosterol. In all other cases the sterol isolated was found to be β-sitosterol.

Ash contains calcium oxide 31.6%, magnesium oxide 7.2%, phosphorus pentaoxide (P_2O_5) 3.6%, and SiO_2 2.7%. A new crystalline compound has been isolated and found to have two glycosides, sennoside A and sennoside B believed to be the laxative principle of senna. Occurance of oxymethyl anthraquinone in fruit upto 1.33% is also reported.

Senna leaves are a sure and safe purgative even for children and weak elderly persons; they are effective in constipation, biliousness, gout and rheumatism, they are given as an infusion, decoction, powder or confection; One of the best preparations of senna is made by infusing two ounces of the leaves and a drachm of ginger in 20 ounces of water in a covered vessel for 15 minutes; half to one ounce of this infusion is taken with hot milk and sugar; another method of taking the leaves is to infuse overnight a dozen leaves in two ounces of water; the strained liquid is taken in the morning on an empty stomach, the leaves may cause nausea and griping and therefore they should be taken with aromatics; senna is also used as an anthelmintic for intestinal worms and as a mild liver stimulant. Senna should not be given in inflammatory conditions of the alimentary canal, fever, piles, menorrhagia, prolapse of the uterus or rectum and pregnancy. A paste of the dried leaves made with vinegar is used for certain skin diseases; the paste is also useful for removing pimples.

Senna pods are used as a purgative, but they are milder and slower in action than the leaves; an infusion made of 4-12 pods in 8 ounces of water is used for adults; but for children and aged the infusion should be made of three to six pods.

Pharmacology

Senna leaves and pods have been used for so long as medicinal agents. Studying the peristaltic activity of senna leaves and their active constituents Straub and Triendl (1937)[7] stated that absorption of active constituents of senna leaves after oral administration was related to the blood supply of the small intestine. Senna substances are active when injected intra-muscularly or intra-venously. There is a latent period of 8 hours 30 minutes between administration and effect on large intestine during which time the glucoside undergo chemical changes with an enzymatic cleavage of anthranol and its oxidation to anthraquinone.

Lloyd W. Hazleton and Kathleen D. Talbert (1945)[8] reported the factors influencing the cathartic activity of senna in mice.

Collier; Fieller; Paris and Bellis (1948)[9] evaluated the purgative activity of senna extacts by comparison of bioassay and chemical assay of senna. The colorimetric method of Kussmaul and Becker gave good agreement with the biological assay of senna. The colorimetric method of Kussmaul and Becker gave good agreement with the biological assay with senna extracts. It was found that chemical assay gives good indication of cathartic activity of any preparation of senna, either freshly made or tested after storage at 45°C for four weeks.

Guillaume Valette (1949)[10] reported the effects of the glycosides of senna (Sennoside A and B) and their hydrolysis products on isolated intestine. They have no effect on isolated guinea pig colon. Both yield rhein on hydrolysis. Rhein produces contraction of the colon. It appears that the anthraquinone glycoside must undergo hydrolysis before they can exert a purgative action.

Lou(1949)[11] stated a bioassay method based upon the number of wet faeces per group of dosed mice applied to senna leaf, senna fruits and extracts of these drugs, pure glycosides (Sennoside A and B) and pure anthracene compounds (aloe - emodin and aloe - emodin anthranol).

Woods, Maribelle and Grote, (1951)[12] repeatedly administered Tinnevelly and Alexandrian senna to mice. Mice showed random variation in laxative action to the same drug when tested week after week but no tolerance developed to either Tinnevelly or Alexandrian senna on repeated administration.

Schmidt (1955)[13] studied the Pharmacology and toxicology of laxatives. The rat was found to be suited to test laxative substances. The substances tested were cascara; aloin; 1,8 dihydroxy anthraquinone; senna glycosides; diacetoxy dipheny lisatin; 4, 4' - dihydroxy triphenyl methane and (4, 4' - dihydroxy diphenyl) (6-methyl - 2 - pyridyl) methane and (4, 4' - dihydroxy diphenyl) (2 - quinolyl) methyl-methane. All drugs tested acted mainly on large intestine but all had a slightly stimulating effect on small intestine as well. Most of the laxatives have acute and chronic toxicity. The margin of therapeutic safety of the synthetic products was better than that of anthraquinone derivatives.

Guillaume Vallete and Marie Louise Hureau (1957)[14] stated the mechanism of senna anthraglucosides actions. They showed that sennosides act directly on smooth muscles of the colon and their binding to the albumin fraction of mucosa proteins is considered.

Seaforth (1962)[15] describes that senna group of plants produces many economical valuable compounds structurally related to new and known drugs. Cassias are best known as Cathartics; some species show antibacterial, antibiotic or furariform activity. Rhein, anthraquinone tannin, chrysin and emodin have been produced in several of the species. Cassias have been used to treat constipation, diabetes and haemoglobin disorders.

The causes of the undesirable side reaction of senna preparations are discussed by Gunther Richter (1966)[16]. These are attributed to overdosage, especially with regard to the higher effect of primary glycosides and also to breakdown products of the sennoside, particularly anthrone glycosides, which irritate the intestinal mucosa.

Fairbairn, and Moss (1970)[17] studied the relative puragative activities of twelve 1, 8-dihydroxy anthracene derivatives including free anthraquinone, anthrone and dianthrone-0-glycosides and they were compared with senna pod power using the production of wet feaces by mice as a criterion of purgation. The higher purgative activity of the dianthrone glycosides was confirmed for the compounds based on rhein. Sennidin (rhein dianthrone) was more active. The results are discussed in relation to the mode of action of orally administered 1, 8-dihydroxy anthracene derivatives.

Garcia, Leng and Ruckebusch (1980)[18] reported the effect of anthraquinone derivatives on rat intestinal motility. Oral administration of oxidized products of Calcium Sennosides to fasted animals increased the increased the activity of the small intestine within two hours. Severe diarrhoea was present 4-6 hours after administration and lasted for about one day. A preparation containing 60% calcium sennoside had a similar but weaker effect. Whereas a preparation containing pure sennoside A and B affected motility only 6-10 hours after oral administration. Intracolonic administration of oxidized products immediately reduced colon motility for 7-8 hours and diarrhoea was present within 40 minutes. Intracolonic calcium sennosides and sennosides A and B induced only small changes in intestinal motility, but diarrhoea also appeared. Thus pure sennosides act predominantly on large intestine motility after their degradation by colonic microorganisms. Oxidized products are already effective in the upper gasrointestinal tract.

Marvola, Koponen and Hiltunen (1981)[19] reported the effect of raw material purity on the acute toxicity and laxative effect of sennosides. In mice, mixtures of pure sennoside A and B and common extracts of senna containing 20-80% sennoside A and B had low toxicities when given orally. However LD_{50} values calculated after intravenous administration (20% extract 171 mg/kg, pure drug 1400 mg/kg) indicated that acute toxicity decreases as the purity of drug increases. The senna extracts were more potent laxatives than the pure drug. Thus common senna preparations contain besides sennoside A and B, compounds with greater toxicity and which have a laxative potency higher than sennosides, or which are synergistic with sennosides.

References

1. Stranb, W. and Gebharadt, H., Arch Expt. Path. Pharmakol. 181, 399, 1936.
2. Chopra, R.N., Nayar, S.L., Chopra, I.C. Glossary of Indian Medicinal plant, C.S.I.R. Publication, 1956.
3. Khorana, M.L., and Sangavi, M.M., J. Pharm Sci. 53(1), 110, 1964.
4. Dane, V.B., Deshmukh, V.K. and Saoji, A.N., Indian J., Pharm., 34, 169, 1972.
5. Chakravarti, R.N., Chakravarti, D., Mitra, M.N., Dasgupta, B., and Maiti, P.C. Bull Cal. Sch. Trop. Med, 3, 163, 1955.
6. Chakravarti, R.N., Chakravarti, D., Dasgupta, B., J. Sci. Ind. Res., 15C, 86, 1956.
7. Straub, W. and Triendl, E., Arch. Exptl. Path. Pharmakol. 185, 1-19, 1937.
9. Collier, H.O.J. Feller E.C., Paris, S.K., and Bellis, D.M., Quart. J. Pharm. Pharmacol 21, 25-9, 1948.
10. Guillaume Valette, Compt. rend. Soc. biol. 143, 74-6, 1949.
11. Lon, T-C., J. Pharm. Pharmacol., 1, 673-82, 1949.
12. Woods, M. Grote, I.W., J. Am. Pharm. Assoc. 40, 198-202, 1951.

13. Schmidt, L., Arch. Exptl. Path. pharmakol., *226*, 207-18, 1955.
14. Guillaume Vallette and Marie, L. H., Therapie, *12*, 885-97, 1957.
15. Seaforth, C.E., Trop. Sci. *4*, 159-62, 1962.
16. Gunther, R., Dent. Apoth. Ztg., *106*(50), 1829-33, 1966
17. Firbairn, J.W., Moss, M.J.R., J. Pharm. Pharmacol, 22(8), 584-93, 1970.
18. Garcia-Villar, R., Leng. Peschlow E (ke, Rukebusch, Y., J. Pharm. Pharmacol., 32(5), 323-9, 1980.
19. Marvola, Martti, Koponen, Arja, Hiltunen, Raimo, Hieltala, Pentti, J. Pharm. Pharmacol., *33*(2), 108-9, 1981.

5
Cassia obtusifolia Linn

Cassia obtusifolia Linn. is Dicotyledonous gymnosperm belonging to Archichlamydeae group in which it belongs to the *order* : Rosales

Sub order : Leguminosineae
Family : Leguminosae
Sub family : Caesalpinaedae
Genera : Cassia, having anthracene derivatives.

Cassia obtusifolia (Fig 5.1, 5.2 and 5.3) is known by different vernacular names in different regions, which are; Bengali-Chakunda, Panevar: English-Fetid Cassia, Ringworm plant; Gujarati-Kawario; Hindi-Chakunda, Panevar; Marathi-Kasodi; Punjabi-Panwar, Pawar; Sanskrit-Avudham, Chakri, Kusuma; Tamil-Senavu, Vindu; Telugu-Tantemu; Urdu-Panwar.

Cassia obtusifolia is an erect, feebly foetid, annual herb, 0.6-2m high. Stems nearly glabrous except glandular hairy young parts. Leaves 7.5-10 cm long; rhachis grooved, more or less pubescent, with a conical gland between the lowest pair of leaflets only; stipules 1.3-2 cm, long linear subulate, caducous. Leaflets 3 pairs, opposite, 2.5-4.5 by 1.3-2 cm (the lowest pair the smallest), obovate-oblong, green, membranous, glabrous or more or less pubescent, base somewhat oblique, usually rounded; main nerves 8-10 pairs; ciliate, appressed, hairy on the lower surface, broadly deltoid at the appex. Petiole 1.5-5 cm long, glandular, hairy along the groove. Flowers usually in subsessile pairs in the axils of the leaves, yellow, 1-2, common peduncle in fruit not exceeding 4 mm long; pedicels 1-2 cm long during anthesis, afterwards elongate up to 4 cm long, calyx glabrous,

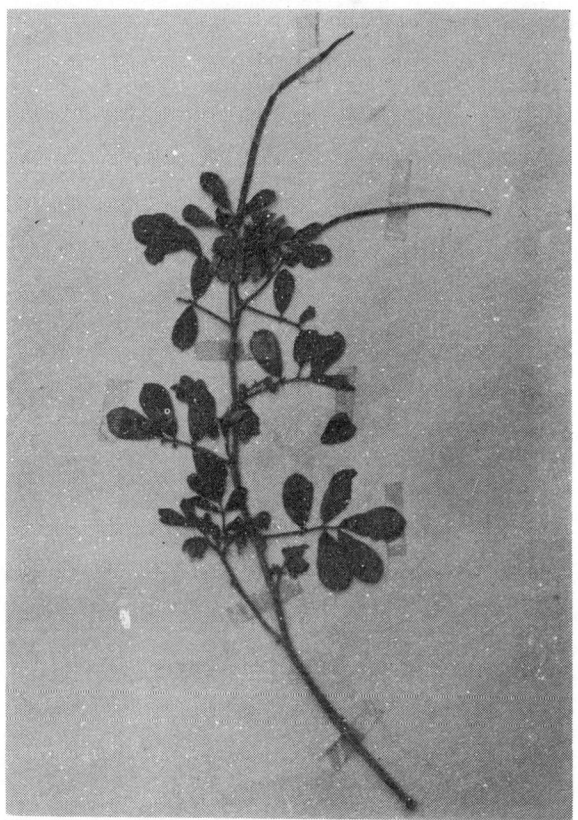

Fig. 5.1 The Plant *Cassia obtusifolia* Linn

divided at the base; segments 6 mm long, ovate acute, spreading. Petals 5, bright yellow, subequal, 1.3.-0.8 cm, oblong, obtuse, the upper petal (standard) truncate. Stamens 10, the 3 upper reduced to minute staminodes, the remaining 7 perfect, subequal. Pods 20-25 by 0.5 cm, subterete, obliquely septate, the sutures broad, valves membranous, glabrous, distinctly transversely reticulated. Seeds 30-35, rhombohedral, 5 mm long, brown, shining. (Fig. 5.4)

Cassia obtusifolia is a very common weed and grows on roadsides, agricultural fields, river beds, forest edges, forest clearings and vacant lots, flowering during rains. The season of the plant is from June-November.

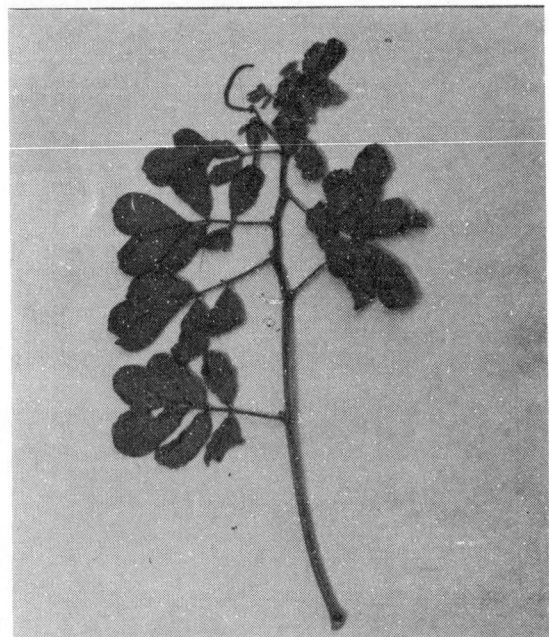

Fig. 5.2 Leaves and Flowers of *Cassia obtusifolia* Linn

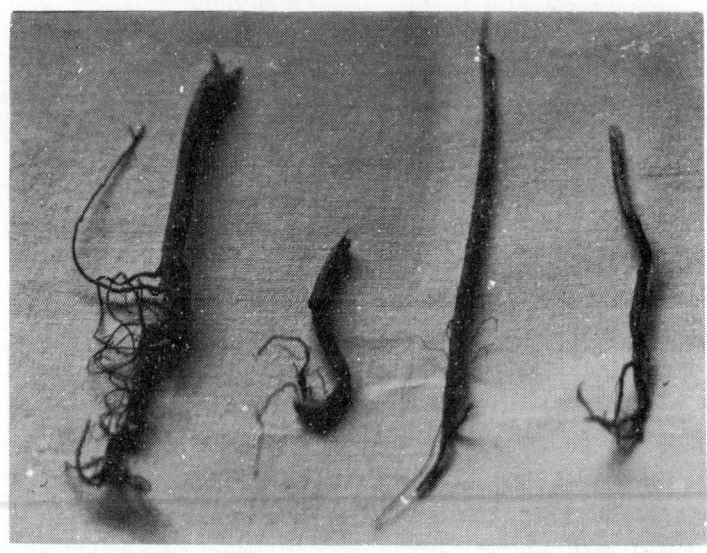

Fig. 5.3 Roots. of *Cassia obtusifolia* Linn

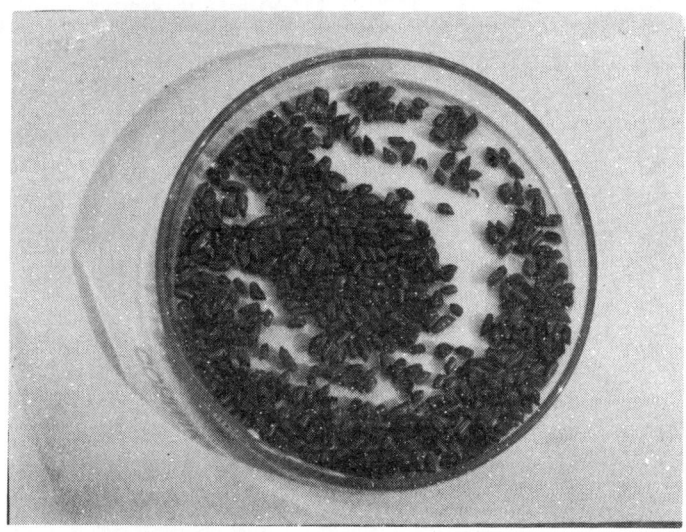

Fig. 5.4 Seeds of *Cassia obtusifolia* Linn

Distribution

Cassia obtusifolia is abundant in Northern, Western and Central India, ascending to 4,000 feet on the West Himalaya; it is found also in Burma and is very common at Singapore. It was introduced originally from tropical America. This plant was long ago recognised by Roxburgh as a species distinct from *Cassia tora* with which it has been united in the Flora of British India. It is often reduced to the synonym of Cassia tora Linn. to which this is closely allied, but this can be distinguished by ciliate sepals, the bottle like necks of the upper 3 anthers, broader areoles of seeds and the presence of a single gland between the first pair of leaflets.

E. PHYTOCHEMICAL AND PHARMACOLOGICAL/BIOLOGICAL INVESTIGATIONS REPORTED ON *CASSIA OBTUSIFOLIA LINN.*

Cassia obtusifolia is a medicinally important plant. Its leaves and roots are used as laxative. Its seeds are called Ketsumeishi in Japan and are used as laxative, tonic and diuretic. This plant has been of immense interest to Indian as well as to foreign research workers. Many research workers investigated this plant:

The following phytochemical work has already been reported on *Cassia obtusifolia* Linn:

Takido[1] (1958) reported chrysophanol, physcion and obtusifolin in the seeds of *Cassia obtusifolia*. In 1960, obtusin (m.p 242-243°C), yellowish brown needles; chryso-obtusin (m.p. 214-215°C), yellow needles and aurantio-obtusin (m.p. 265-266°C) were isolated from the seeds of *Cassia obtusifolia*[2]. The structures of these pigments were established respectively as 1,6,7-trimethoxy-2,8-dihydroxy-3-methyl anthraquinone. 1,6,7,8-tetra methoxy-2-hydroxy-3-methyl anthraquinone and 1,7-dimethoxy-2,6,8-trihydroxy-3-methyl anthraquinone.

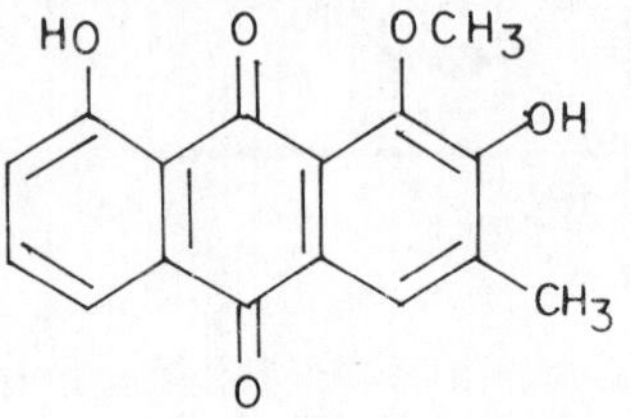

Obtusifolin

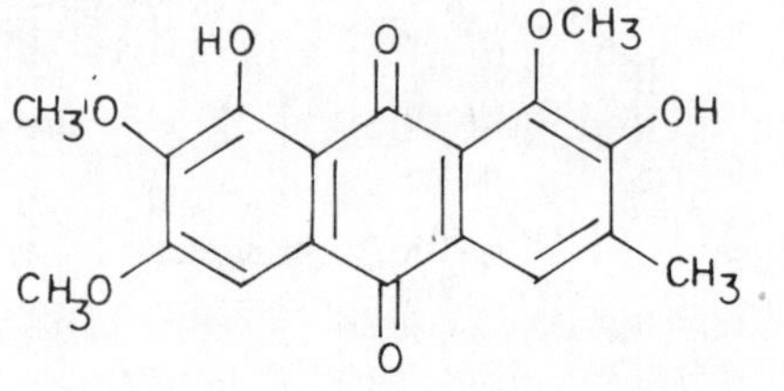

Obtusin

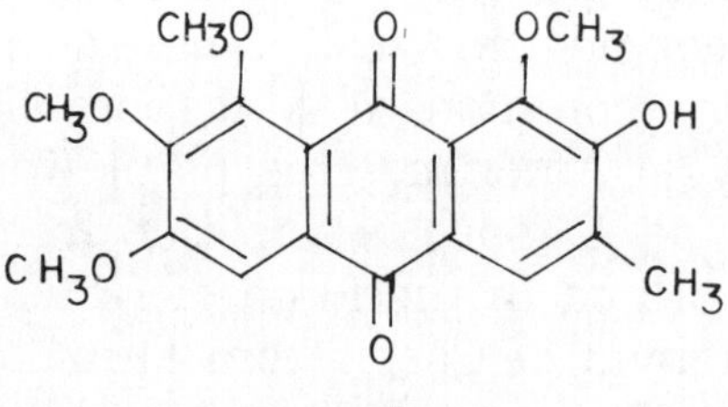

Chryso-obtusin

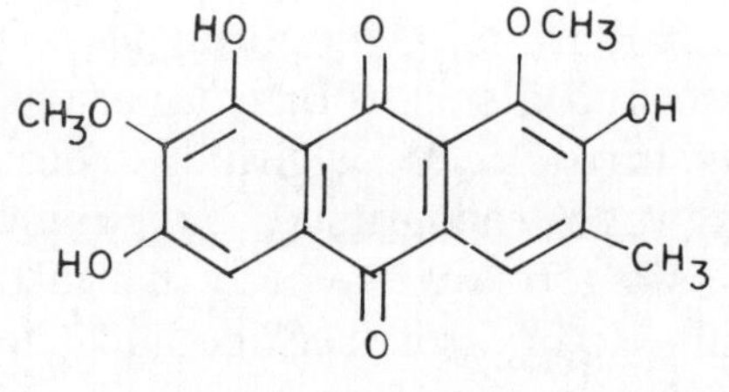

Aurantio-obtusin

Kapur and Pant (1963) analysed the plant for total soluble carbohydrate and qualitatively by paper chromatography for individual soluble carbohydrate in *Cassia obtusifolia* was 5.56%.

Takido and Takahashi[3] (1964) isolated gluco-obtusifolin and gluco aurantio-obtusin from the seeds of *Cassia obtusifolia* by column chromatography. Gluco-obtusifolia (m.p. 205-206°C) gave a brown colour with ferric chloride, red with 5% sodium carbonate and orange with ethanolic solution of magnesium acetate. Glucoaurnatio-obtusin (m.p. 242-243°C) $C_{23}H_{24}O_{12}$, pale yellow, showed the same color reactions as gluco-obtusifolin.

Kimura *et.al.*[4] (1966) isolated a new glucoside, cassiaside, pale yellow micro needles, m.p. 256-257°C, $C_{20}H_{20}O_{10}$ from the methanolic extracts of the seeds by column chromatography. It gave one mole of nor-rubrofusarin and one mole of glucose and its permethyl ether afforded 5,8-di-O-methyl-nor-rubrofusarin by hydrolysis with 5% hydrochloric acid. Thus the structure of cassiaside has been established as nor-rubrof usarin-6-β-mono-D-Gluco-side.

Cassia obtusifolia and *Cassia tora* have received confused treatment by taxonomists, being regarded by some as synonyms while by others as distinct species. Subramaniam[5] (1968) showed that *Cassia obtusifolia* L. and *Cassia tora* L. are two distinct taxa. Two species can not be the same from biochemical evidence obtained from a study of chemical components of their seeds. The seeds of *Cassia tora* L. contain rubrofusarin and non rubrofusarin which belong to the class of naphthopyrones while the seeds of *Cassia obtusifolia* L. contain closely related compounds chrysophanol, physcion, obtusin, obtusifolin, chryso-obtusin and aurantio-obtusin all of which are anthraquinones and chemically these groups are different. Singh[6] (1968) also presented some convincing experimental evidence from ecological studies of *Cassia tora* L. and *Cassia obtusifolia* L. to indicate that these are two distinct taxa.

Radha Pant *et.al.*[7]. (1974) analysed seeds of *Cassia obtusifolia* for its free amino acid composition. Wild leguminous seeds of *Cassia obtusifolia* were collected, powdered 100 mesh in a hand grinder and stored in air tight bottles. Seeds powder was defatted with petroleum ether (60°-80oC) in a Soxhlet extractor. Extraction and isolation of free amino acids from seed powder was made by stirring the defatted seed powder (1 gm) with warm ethanol (10 ml, 70% V/V) for 30 minutes. After centrifugation the residue was re-extracted with ethanol, centrifuged, and two supernatants combined. This process was repeated (8-9 times) till the supernatant was negative to Ninhydrin test. The pooled supernatant was then evaporated to dryness in vacuo, dissolved in distilled water (0.5-1 ml,) centrifuged and the clear supernatant(2-10 μl) was employed for qualitative free amino acid analysis by paper partition chromatography on Whatman No.1 filter paper sheets. Free amino acids were detected by two-dimensional technique of Datta, Dent and Harris employing phenol (80% W/V)- ammonia and butanol; acetic acid:water (4:1:5) as developing solvents. Chromatograms after development were sprayed with ninhydrin (0.1% W/V) in butanol. Identity of various amino acids was confirmed by using specific spray reagents.

Essential amino acid content of non edible leguminous seeds of Cassia obtusifolia (results expressed as gm amino acid/16 gm N) Histidine-2.8; Lysine-6.5; Methionine-0.6; Ph, alanine-2.8; Tyrosine-1.63; Ph.alanine + tyrosine - 4.43; Leucine + Isoleucine-7.1; Valine-2.3; Threonine-2.9.

Koshioka and Takino[8] (1978) established a method of quantitative estimation of anthraquinones in *Cassia obtusifolia* seeds, and the change of anthraquinone contents in the seeds of *Cassia obtusifolia* Linn. with various grades of maturity and aging was studied. Quantitative estimations of anthraquinones in samples obtained from various places were made. The absorbance of the alkaline extract after treatment with 5% sodium hydroxide solution containing 2% ammonia was measured at 520 mm, using 1,8-dihydroxy anthraquinone as a standard. The optimum time for measurement was 60-180 minutes after the completion of alkaline extraction and the optimum time for hydrolysis was 75 minutes. As maturity of the seeds progressed, the amount of free anthraquinones decreased and the amount of bound anthraquinones increased gradually although the total amount was constant. The content of free anthraquinoness was 0.01%-1.29% and total contents varied 1.04-1.31%. The crude drug obtained from different places might be classified into two groups according to content of anthraquinones.

Matsuura[9] (1978) isolated triacontan-1-ol, stigmasterol, β-sitosletrol, β-D glucoside, friedelin, palmitic acid, stearic acid, succinic acid, d-tartaric acid, uridine, myo-inositol, d-ononitol, Kaempferol, quercetin, juglanin, astragalin, quercitrin and iso quercitrin from the leaves of *Cassia obtusifolia*.

Kitanaka and Takido[10] (1981) isolated torosachrysone and two new naphthalenic lactones, isotoralactone and cassialactone from seeds of *Cassia obtusifolia*. Yellow prisms, m.p. 196-200°C, $C_{16}H_{16}O_5$ was identified as torosachrysone by direct-comparison with an authentic sample. Isotoralactone, pale yellow needles, m.p. 233-235°C, $C_{15}H_{12}O_5$, gave a positive ferric chloride reaction and with Gibbs reagent gave a fluorescent light blue under

U.V. radiation. Cassialactone, very pale yellow needles, m.p. 196-197.5°C, $C_{16}H_{16}O_6$ was ligh pink under U.V. radiation and gave positive ferric chloride and Gibbs tests. Biogenetically cassialactone may be derived from torosachrysone by a Baeyer-Villiger type oxidation.

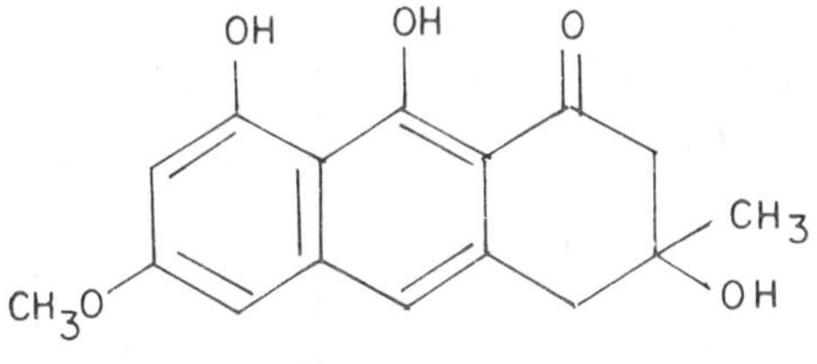

Torosachrysone

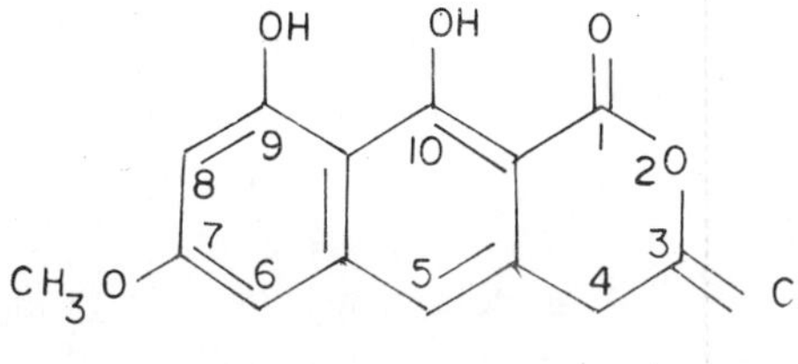

Isotoralactone

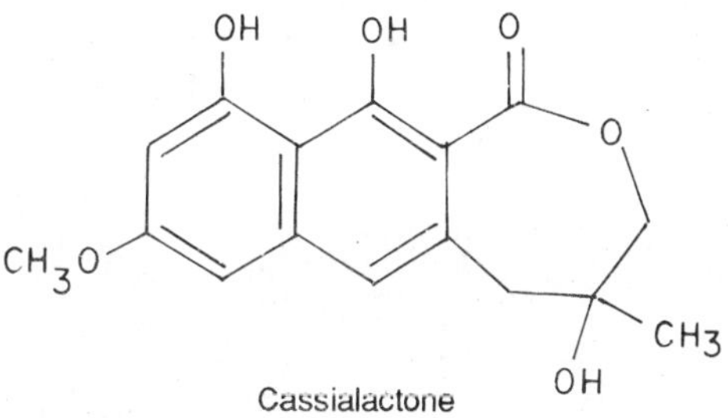

Cassialactone

Yashui and Ohno[11] (1982) examined the distribution of D-(+) -ononitol (I) and galactosyl ononitol (II) in seeds of *Cassia obtusifolia* by gas chromatography. The seeds showed existence of (I) and (II) at 0.05-0.22% and 0.03-0.23% respectively.

Kitanaka and Takido[12] (1984) reported three new anthraquinones, 1-desmethyl chryso-obtusin (I), I-desmethylobtusin (II) and 1-desmethyl aurantio-obtusin (III), along with chrysophanol-10, 10'-bianthrone, questin and benzoic acid in seeds of *Cassia obtusifolia* and their structures were established on the basis of spectral and chemical evidence. Chrysophanol-10, 10' -bianthrone, yellow needles, (m.p.221°C) was identified by direct comparison with a synthetically prepared sample.

Questin, Yellow needles (m.p. 300-303°C) $C_{16}H_{12}O_6$ and benzoic acid, colorless plates (m.p. 121-124°C) $C_7H_6O_2$ were identified by direct comparison with authentic samples. The three new anthraquinone derivatives (compounds I-III) having vicinal -OH groups showed a purple color in methanolic magnesium acetate.

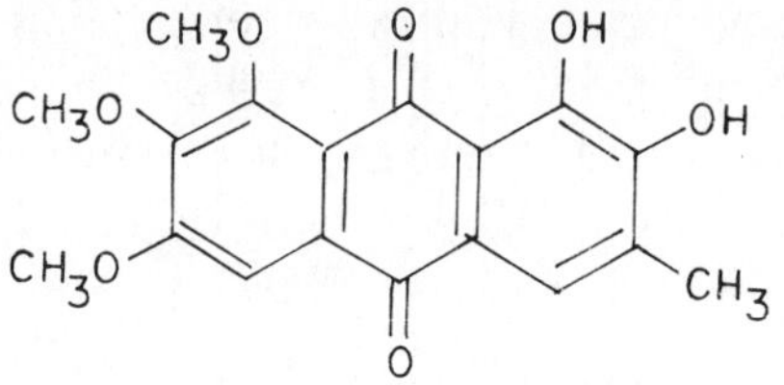

1-desmethyl chryso-obtusin
(I)

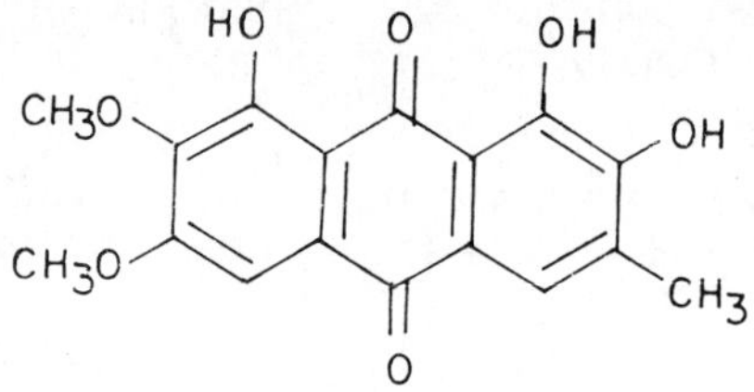

1-desmethyl obtusin
(II)

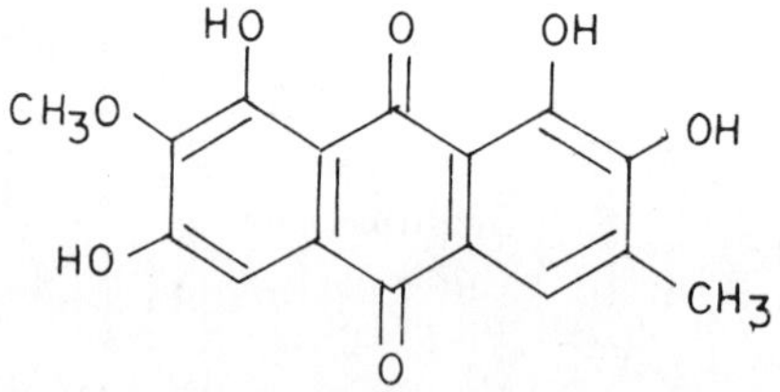

1-desmethyl aurantio-obtusin
(III)

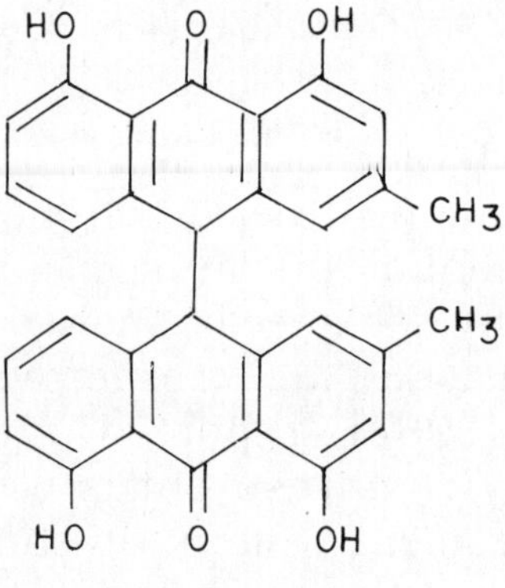

Chrysophanol-10, 10' bianthrone

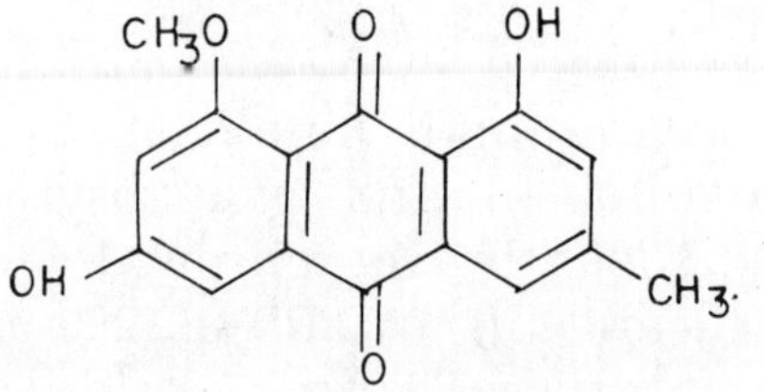

Questin

Kitanaka *et.al.*[13] (1985) reported two new anthraquinones alaternin 1-O-β-D-glucopyranoside and chryso-obtusin 2-O-β-gluco pyranoside, along with physcion 8-O-<98>-D-glucopyranoside from the seeds of *Cassia obtusifolia* and their structures were established on the basis of spectral and chemical evidence.

In 1986, nine anthraquinones (islandicin, helminthosporin, chrysophanol, physcion, xanthorin, 8-O- methyl chrysophanol, obtusifolin, emodin and aloe-emodin), a naphtho-β-pyrone (rubrofusarin), a benzoquinone (2,5-dimethoxy benzoquinone), phytosterols and betulinic acid were isolated from the roots of *Cassia obtusifolia*[14]. Compounds benzoquinone (2,5-dimethoxy benzoquinone) and aloe-emodin, isolated from the roots and isotoralactone, toralactone, question and torosachrysone from the seeds showed antimicrobial activities.

The following uses and pharmacological/biological work has already been reported on the *Cassia obtusifolia* Linn.

Cassia obtusifolia is reputed for its medicinal value in Ayurvedic and Unani system of medicine. Kirtikar and Basu[120] reported many uses of *Cassia obtusifolia*. The root is useful for skin diseases, tuburculous glands and ringworm. The leaves are bitter with a sharp taste and some flavour; hot, dry, digestible, refrigerant, anthelmintic, antipyretic, laxative, diuretic; cure bronchitis, asthma, leprosy, skin disease, piles, itching, head troubles, "tridosha", urinary discharges, useful in diseases of the heart and in ringworm. The fruit and seeds are anthelmintic, astringent to the bowels, cure tumours, leprosy, skin diseases, scabies, cough, asthma and burning sensation (Ayurveda). The leaves are laxative; useful in indolent ulcers, leprosy, skin diseases. The seeds are demulcent and maturant; useful in itch, ulcers, ringworm, skin diseases (Unani).

The leaves are gently aperient; fried in castor oil, they are considered a good application to foul ulcers. The seeds ground with sour buttermilk are used to ease the irritation of itchy eruptions; and the root, rubbed on a stone with lime juice, is supposed to be one of the best remedies for ringworm. The leaves are also used as a poultice to hasten suppuration. A warm ready in gout, sciatica and pains in the joints.

In Indo China, the pods are used in dysentery and ophthalmia. In the Malay Peninsula, the seeds are used internally and externally for all sorts of eye diseases, preparations of the seeds are also given for liver complaints and boils.

In Madagascar and La Reunion, the plant is considered antihysteric, and febrifuge.

An oil named "Chakramardha" whose chief ingredients are *Cassia obtusifolia* and *Eclipta alba* was used in cases of ringworm as an external application and found to be very beneficial (Koman).

Charaka recommended the fruit in snake-bite, the bark and the roots in scorpion-sting. According to Mhaskar and Cains fruit is useless in the treatment of snake-bite; the roots and bark are equally useless for scorpion-sting.

The leaves are cheapest and unparalleled remedy for "Half-headache"[15]. This plant has the natural character of opening of leaves at sunrise and clasping at sunset. Half headache also starts in morning at sunrise and increases with the heat of sun rays and decreases after mid-day and in the evening it totally disappears and so the disease has its local or Hindi name as `Kirnwah' and the following is the best remedy for this disease;

Early in the morning about an hour before sunrise, take 10-15 leaves of *Cassia obtusifolia* with one tola of Gur, chew and eat them with one glass of water, the half-headache is sure to disappear the same day and if some trouble still, remains repeat it the next day and see the magic effect of the leaves the disease will totally disappear.

Poultices are made by pounding the leaves with rice for skin complaints and the leaves may be rubbed on the face of a child to induce sleep[16] The plant has also been tried as a green manure[17,18].

Mukadam[19] (1976) reported the antifungal activity in deproteinised leaf extracts of *Cassia obtusifolia*, Spore germination of *Alternaria brassicicola*, *Helminthosporium apattarnae*, *Pestalotia* species, *Penicillium purpurogenum*, *Aspergillus niger*, *Trichothecium* species, *Neurospora* species, *Fusarium* species, *Trichoderma* species and *Rhizopus* species was used to assess antifungal activity.

In 1978, occurrence of fungus, *Pseudocerco sporanigricans* on *Cassia obtusifolia* was reported for the first time in India[20]. Small circular to irregular light brown spots, 5-9 mm in size were observed on both the surfaces of the living leaves of almost all the parts of *Cassia obtusifolia* Linn. at Modinagar, Microscopic examination of the infected portions revealed the presence of fungus.

Singh *et.al.*[21] (1979) studied the hypoglycaemic and hypocholesterolemic effect of *Cassia obtusifolia* seeds. The mean value of total blood cholesterol of fasted young albino rats maintained on laboratory stocked diet was found to be 205.73 ± 11.24 mg/100 ml. Maximum lowering effect in total blood cholesterol level was 13.64%. In diabetic albino rats which were fed on experimental diet consisting of *Cassia obtusifolia* seeds for 15 days, there was insignificant decrease in blood sugar level by 2.09% and also in blood cholesterol level by 3,24%.

Nikaido *et.al.*[22] (1981) reported the inhibitory effect of seeds of *Cassia obtusifolia* on cyclic AMP phosphodiesterase. Cyclic AMP phospho-diesterase has been used as a screening tool for the detection of biologically active substances. correlation between pharmacological activity in vivo and inhibition of phosphodiesterase in vitro has been reported. Reproducible inhibition was shown in two successive tests each carried out in duplicate. Extracts which showed inhibition in screening test were further fractionated into chloroform soluble and insoluble fractions to clarify the solubilities of inhibitors. Choloroform soluble fractions showed higher activity than the corresponding chloroform insoluble fractions, indicating that the inhibitors were soluble in organic solvent.

Cassia obtusifolia has been reported as new host for *Sclerotium rolfsii* from tarai belt North Eastern Uttar Pradesh[23].

In 1986, *Cassia obtusifolia* was screened for its inhibitory effect on adenosine 5'-diphosphate (ADP), arachidonic acid (AA) or collagen induced rat platelet aggregation. The results suggested that *Cassia obtusifolia* is a potential source of inhibitors of platelet aggregation[24].

Kitanaka and Takido[14] (1986) reported antimicrobial activity of seeds and roots of *Cassia obtusifolia*. Compounds benzoquinone (2,5-dimethoxy-benzoquinone) and aloe-emodin isolated from the roots and isotoralactone, toralactone, questin and torosachrysone from the seeds showed antimicrobial activities.

The tissue culture work is also reported on *Cassia obtusifolia*[25]. The plant hormonal requirements for the tissue culture of *Cassia obtusifolia* to find an optimal conditions for the callus formation were studied under correlation with formation of anthraquinone pigments, which was detected by dual-wavelength TLC Zig Zag scanning. Differentiation of callus tissues induced from *Cassia obtusifolia* occurs depending on the ratio of IAA and cytokinins in the culture medium. From the callus tissues obtained by the optimum condition for callus formation (dry weight : 11.48 gm from 15 flasks) chloroform extract (0.12 gm) was prepared, which was separated into 8 fractions by the preparative layer chromatography. The anthraquinonic pigments produced by the callus tissues were thus identified in comparison with authentic samples by their m.p., TLC, I.R. and Mass spectra. Obtusin and chryso-obtusin which are contained in the seeds of *Cassia obtusifolia* were not found in the callus tissues of the plant. Emodin, aloe-emodin, islandicin and xanthorin have not been reported as the constituents of the seeds, while they have been isolated from the callus tissue.

References

1. Takido, M., *Chem. Pharm. Bull*, 1958, 6, 397.
2. Radha, P., Kapur, A.S., *Naturwissenschaften*, 1963, 50, 95.
3. Takido, M., Takahashi, S., *Shoyakugaku Zasshi*, 1964,17, 43.
4. Kimura, Y., Takido, M. and Takahashi, S., *Yakugaku Zasshi*, 1966, 86, 1087.
5. Subramanian, S.S, *Curr. Sci*, 1968, 37(17), 493.
6. Singh, J.S., Curr, Sci, 1968, 13, 381.
7. Radha, P., Nair, C. Rajagopalan, Singh, S.K., Koshti, G.S. *Curr. Sci*, 1974, 43(8), 325.
8. Koshioka, M., Takino, Y, *Chem. Pharm. Bull*, 1978, 26(5), 1343.
9. Matsuura, S., *Yakugaku Zasshi*, 1978, 98(9), 1288.
10. Kitanaka, S., Takido, M., *Phytochemistry*, 1981, 20(8), 1951.
11. Yashui, T., Ohno, S., *Nippon Nogei Kagaku Kaishi*, 1982, 56(11), 1053.
12. Kitanaka, S., Takido, M., *Chem, Pharm. Bull*, 1984, 32(3), 860.
13. Kitanaka, S. Kimura, F., Takido, M. *Chem. Pharm. Bull*, 1985, 33(3), 1275.
14. Kitanaka, S. Takido, M., *Yakugaku Zasshi*, 1986, 106(4), 302.
15. Kirtikar and Basu, *Indian Medicinal Plants*, Vol.II (2nd Ed.) 1933, 865.
16. Srivastava, S.P., *Indian For.*, 1956, 82(1), 49.

17. Burkill and Haniff Gard. Bull, 1930, 6, 194.
18. Heyne, K. Nutt. Plant Med. Ind. Ed. 1927, pp. 745.
19. Mukadam, D.S. *Ind.J. Microbiol*, 1976, 16(2), 78.
20. Dube, V.P., *Curr. Sci*, 1978, 47(23), 913.
21. Singh, K.N., Misra, V., *Med. and Surg*, 1979, 19, 8.
22. Nikaido, T., Ohmoto, T., Noguchi, H., Kinoshita, T., Saitoh. H., Sankawa, U., *Planta Medica*, 1981, 43(1), 18.
23. Rai, A.N., Singh, S.K., Kamal, *Environ. India*, 1982, 5(I & II), 55.
24. Yun-Choi, H.S, Kim, J.H. Lee, J.R. *Korean J. Pharmacog.*, 1986, 17(1), 19.
25. Takahashi, S., Kitanaka, S., Takido. M., Ebizuka Y., Sankawa, U., Hoson, M., Kobayashi, M., Shibata, S., *Planta. Medica*, 1978, 33, 389.

6
Dolichos biflorus Linn

GENUS DOLICHOS

Dolichos is a well known and wide spread genus of the family Leguminoseae occuring mainly in the tropical countries It contains most of the edible beans and many pulses.

The major Indian species of Dolichos (besides D. biflorus are: [1,2]

Dolichos lablab	: (Flat bean, Hyacinth bean) Hindi : 'Sem'
Dolichos bulbuosus	:
Dolichos catjang	: (Cowpea, Cow gram) Hindi : 'Lobia'
Dolichos cylindricus	:
Dolichos fabaeformis	:
Dolichos falacatus	:
Dolichos lignosus	
Dolichos minimus	
Dolichos tranquelanicus	
Dolichos trilobatus	
Dolichos pruriens	: (Cowhedge) Hindi : 'Kavach'
Dolichos sesban	
Dolichos soja (Soyabean)	

Many of these have traditional medicinal uses in Ayurveda Those listed by Nadkarni[1] are:

Dolichos catiang	: Diuretic
Dolichos fabaeformis	: Diuretic
Dolichos falacatus	: Roots used in piles, constipation. ophthalmia and skin diseases.

	Decoction of seeds is used in rheumatism. Experimental analgesic and antitumor activity observed[3,4]
Dolichos lablab	: Seeds are aphrodisiac and also used to stop nose bleeding and in phlegmatic disorder. Root is poisonous.
Dolichos minimus	: Seeds are Poisonous.
Dolichos trilobatus	: Leaves are used as laxative
Dolichos pruriens	: Seeds are used as astringent, anthelmrntic, nerve tonic and aphrodisiac. Seeds are used also in Leucorrhoea, sprmatonhea profuse menstruation and paralysis. Roots are used as nerve tonic in facial paralysis, hemiplegia, delirium due to cholera and other fevers, root paste is applied to reduce dropsy and elephantitis. Infusion of pods is administered in dropsy. Pod hair are locally stimulant and mild vesicant and used as vermifuge.
Dolichos sesban	: Seeds and bark are astringent and used in diarrhoea, in checking excess menstruation, skin eruptions and itch. They also reduce enlarged spleen. Leaf poultice is used in reducing boils, abcesses, hydrocele and inflammatory rheumatic swellings.

All the other species are used either as human food (Beans or seeds or as animal fodder (leaves and stem). Some of the other important species of Dolichos (not found in India) are:

Dolichos tonkinensis	: Nutritive (Africa)[5]
Dolichos sinensis	: Nutritive [6]
Dolichos axillaris	
Dolichos debilis	
Dolichos formosus	: Nutritive and fodder[7]
Dolichos densiflora	
Dolichos jacquini	: Human phytoprecipitins in seeds[8]

Dolichos sericus
Dolichos trilobatus   : rglutamyl phenyl alanine in seeds
Dolichos glabrescens   : chemotaxonomically important[9,10]
Dolichos marginata   : Pterocarpinoids from bark[11]
Dolichos
  kilimandscharius   : Fungicidal and Molluscicidal
                             saponins.[12]

DOLICHOS BIFLORUS LINN - MORPHOLOGY (Fig. 6.1 & 6.2)

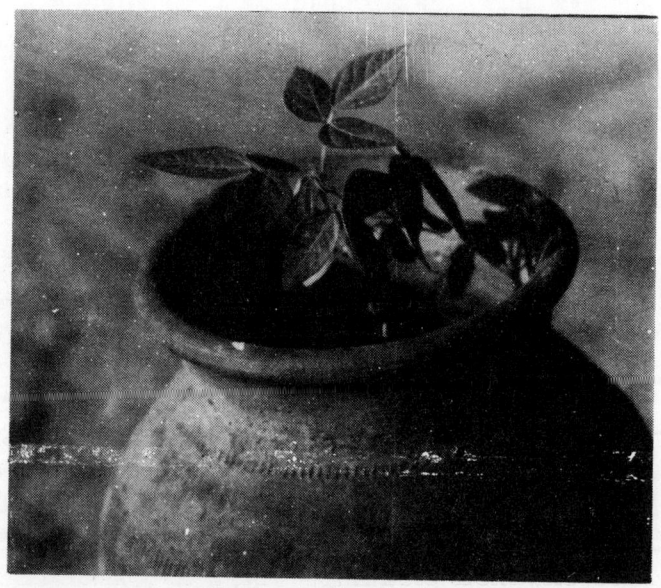

Fig. 6.1 *Dolichos biflorus* (white seed variety) grown in a pot

Family   : Leguminoseae (Papillionaceae)
Sanskrit   : 'Kulattha'
Hindi   : 'Kulthi'
Bengali   : 'Kurti-kalai', 'Kulattha-kalai'
Marathi   : 'Koolthi'
Gujarati   : 'Kulti', 'Kulit'
Konkani   : 'Kulithu'
Telegu   : 'Ulavelu'
Tamil   : 'Kollu'
Kannada   : 'Huruli'

Malayalam	:	'Kullu', 'Mutira'
English	:	Horse-gram
French	:	Dolic-a-deux

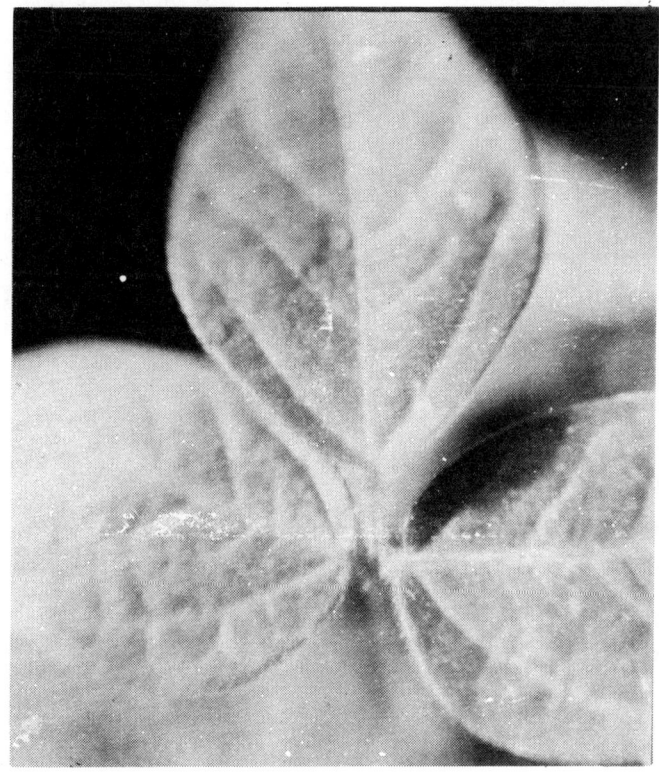

Fig. 6.2 *Dolichos biflorus* (white seed variety-leaflets)

Oliver[7] describes *Dolichos biflorus* Linn as:

Stems very wide climbing, slender, slightly pubescent, oblong blunt, subglabrescent leaflets on a petiole, lateral ones very unequal sided, stipullae minute and linear. Flowers 1-3 on very short pedicels in the axils of the leaves. Calyx slightly downy with upper teeth quite connate, the side lanceolate and the lowest one linear. Corolla yellow. Pod linear, subsessile, nearly straight, glabrous, 6-8 seeded, tipped with a persistant style.

The Dictionary of Economic Products (DEP)[13] and the **Flora** of British India[14] describes *Dolichos biflorus* Linn as:

A branched suberect or trailing annual, with small trifoliate leaves, bearing, when mature, narrow, flat, curved pods, 1.5" to 2" long tipped with a persistant style. The pods contain 5-6 flattened ellipsoid seeds, 1/8" - 1/4" long. (Fig. 6.3)

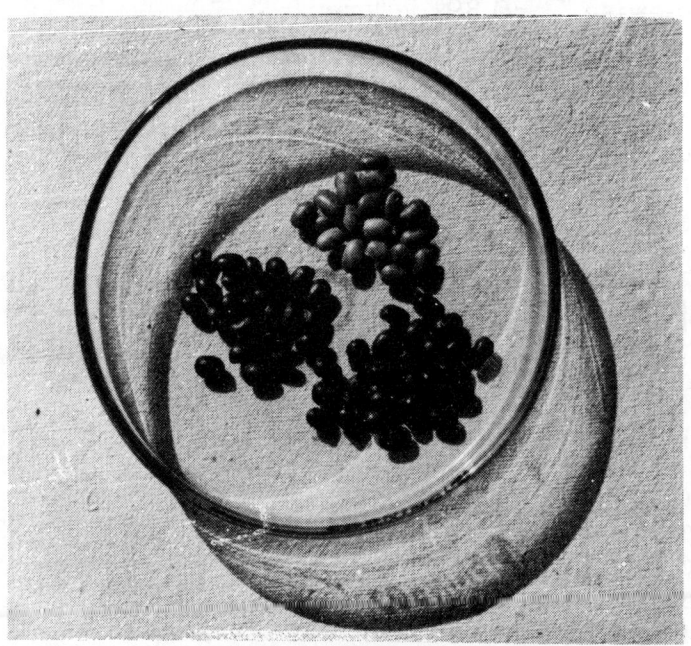

Fig. 6.3 *Dolichos biflorus* seeds showing three different varieties

Several agricultural varieties are available and they are often commercially available as mixture of seeds. 5 strains of 'Kulthi' have been studied and characterized morphologically and biochemically by Chattopadyay *et.al.*[15]

Seeds treated with different doses of x-rays and ethyl-methane sulfonate, change seed colour from black brown mottled to light brown.[16]

PHYTOCHEMICAL COMPOSITIONS OF DOLICHOS BIFLORUS LINN

The seed analysis as compiled in the Wealth of India[17] is:

Moisture   : 11.8%
Crude Protein : 22.0%
Fat   : 0.5%

Minerals   : 3.1%
Fibres   : 5.3%
Carbohydrates   : 57.3%
Calcium   : 0.28%
Phosphorus   : 0.39%
Iron   : 0.0076%
Nicotinic acid : 0.0015%
Carotene   : 119Iµ/100gms.
Arginine   : 6.0-7.1% of total Nitrogen
Tyrosine   : 6.68% of total Nitrogen
Lysine   : 7.64% of total Nitrogen

Enzyme urease was first detected by Mateer and Marshall 18 in 1916 in the seeds of *Dolichos biflorus*. Menon and Rao[19] presented it as a new and cheap source of urease in 1932. Venkatasubban *et.al.*[20]. found that germinated seeds gave higher urease activity than the ungerminated seeds, which, they proposed, indicated that germination merely increases the solubility of enzyme. Damodaran *et.al.*[21] suggested arginine as the precursor of the amides, 28-50% of which was urea[22]. However only a part of urea arise from the hydrolysis of arginine, which suggested that rapid mobilization of urease also helped in urea accumulation in the germinated seedlings. Much later in 1981 Criease from *Dolichos biflorus* was characterized and 4% of urease was obtained from the seeds which was half active as the Merck Product.[23]

Proteins and Amino acids from *D. biflorus* have been extensively studied. In 1930, Narayana[24] found out that the globulin contains sufficient quantities of Arginine, Tyrosine and Lysine but deficient in Cysteine and Tryptophan. Rapid solubilization of reserve protein in the early stages of germination was detected by Damodaran *et.al.*[21] with soluble nitrogen reaching up to 90% of the total nitrogen within the first 24 hours. This amount decreased somewhat because of resynthesis into insoluble proteins but remained between 70-80% for a few weeks. Arginine disappeared rapidly with aging of the seedling with increase of amides. Asparagine was detected in good quantities in the germinating seeds[25]. Bagchi *et.al.*[26] separated and identified free amino acids Aspartic acid, Lysine, Phenylalanine, Glycine, Threonine, Alanine, Tyrosine, Valine, Glutamic acid, Leucine, Proline, Serine and Tryptophan by paper chromatography.

Histidine was found absent. 2-D paper chromatography on seeds showed rapid increase of Arginine just after germination.[27] Seeds were found deficient in Methionine and Cystiene. The root nodules containing a Nitrogen fixing bacteria[28], contained a mixture of free amino acids with the main components as Asparagine, Glycine, Alanine, Valine, Leucine, a-amino- butyric acid, a-amino-butyric acid, Arginine and Tyrosine.[29] Grown under tropical conditions the seeds were reported to be higher in essential Amino acids content except Cysteine, Methionine and Tryptophan.[30] During germination Amino acids increased due to increased protease action and proline increased due to decreased proline dehydrogenase activity[31]. Salt stress by 100 meq/l of Nacl and Na_2SO_4 caused increased activity of nitrate reductase, alanine-amino-transferase, aspartate-amino-transferase, glutamate dehydrogenase and gultamine synthetase[32]. This study explained to some extent the amino acids profile changes during the germination.

Niyogi et.al.[33] determined that the seeds were highly nutritive with 10% protein intake in rats. However Ray[34] found out that autoclaved seeds were better due to destruction of a trypsin inhibitor. Protein components as determined by Pant et.al.[35] : Crude protein:25% in which globulins 63-83%, Albumin-3.5-15.4%, Glutein-2.8-6.8% and Prolamine 0-2%. Non protein nitrogen content was 4.7.-7.0% of total nitrogen. Amino acids content of the seed protein was determined by Manage and Sohonie[36] as: Tryptophan-63% Methionine Cysteine-48%, Threonine-65%, Valine-77% and Isoleucine-89% of the same in egg protein. High Lysine and Phenyl alanine contents were determined in the protein.[37, 38] Mean protein content, as determined by Begum et.al.[39] was 23.12 gm%. Singh and Bird[40] isolated haemagglutinins exhibiting absolute specificity for human blood group A and predominantly for subgroup A_1,[41] from the seeds in 1956. This haemagglutinin or lactin was purified electrophoretically[42] and later patented[43]. The agglutinin isolated by fractionation and chromatography was characterized by Kuehnemund et.al.[44]. as a glycoprotein of molecular weight about 130000 with amino acids and carbohydrates (0.5% galactose, 0.2% mannose, rhamnose and fructose). The lectin was further purified by Etzler et.al.[45] and it showed exclusive agglutinating action on group A_1 erythrocytes[46]. Manage et.al.[47] found that the agglutinin was non toxic to rats and mice-whereas that from Dolichos lablab had 4 identical subunits of the lectin with alanine at the N terminal. Thy were isolated by Pere et.al.[48] and later on characterised by Carter et.al.[49,50]. Amino acids sequences of the subunits I and II, determined by Etzler et.al.[51] were identical. Number of receptors for this lectin on human erythrocyte membrane was determined to be about 6×10^5 sites/cell which were distinct from other lectin receptors[52]. A cross reactive material to the seed lectin autibodies were isolated from the leaves and systems by Talbot et.al.[53] and later characterised[54]. A radioimmunoassay for the lectins was developed by them later[55]. It was found by Loreutz et.al.[56] that, the lectins react at very low intensity with the enzymes-Arylamidase, Alkaline Phosphatase, -glutanyl-transferase, and cholinesterase of human serum-with formation of active but insoluble complexes. Lectins involvement in the higher plant-fungus interaction was hinted at by Etzler[57] and later distribution and properties of the lectin like glycoproteins from leaves and stems and their physiological significances were reviewed by her[58]. A new and non specific lectin was isolated and partially characterised by Handa et.al.[59] Quinn[60] isolated and characterised a root lectin and studied in vivo biosynthesis of the seed lectin by photo affinity labelling. Schnell and Etsler[61] isolated a lectin from the leaves and stems which showed 84% homology to the seed lectin amino acids sequence and they proposed that they are encoded by differentially expressed genes evolved to carry out tissue specific functions. Schnell[62] later determined the molecular origin and primary structure of the two differentially expressed lectins. Recently radiolabelling experiments have indicated Methionine and Glucosanine to be the precursors in lectin biosynthesis.[63]

Various plant enzymes, besides urease, have been isolated from *Dolichos biflorus*. Bheemeshwar et.al.[64] detected small amounts of ribonuclease in 1950. Mukundan et.al.[65] isolated Nicotinamide deaminase from the cotyledons. Meyer et.al.[66] isolated and purified, b-N-acetylglucosaminidase, a & b-galactosidase, a-mannosidase and b-glucosidase from germinating seeds. An unusual Allantoinase was detected and purified by Mary and Sastry[67]. Mehta et.al.[68] detected and isolated an inhibitor of trypsin and chymotrypsin which are thought to be responsible for the non-bioavailability of the proteins of the uncooked seeds. Activities of strach phosphorylase and protease during germination was studied by Sudhakar and coworkers[69].

The seeds as well as the vegetative body are rich in vitamins. Makhijani and Banerjee[70] extracted about 100 mg of carotene from a kg of the straw. Sohonie and Misra[71] extracted Nicotinic acid from the seeds, Dakshinamurthi extracted[72] choline (0.189%) and Chitre et.al.[73] detected Thiamine and Riboflavine. Thiamine content was correlated with the tissue growth during germination by Iengar et.al.[74] and Pant et.al.[75] detected Riboflavine increase in the germinating and long stored seeds. Role of Thiamine in root and shoot growth was estimated by Sastry et.al.[76] Tocopherol was determined in the seeds by Nazir and Megar[77]. The seeds and the straw nave a high mineral content, the total content varying from 2.2 to 3.3% of the dry weight[78]

Calcium	:	0.191-0.43%[79]
Phosphate	:	0.244-0.465%
Ca:PO$_4$ ratio	:	1:1-1:1.9
Iron	:	0.013-0.071%
Molybdenum	:	1 ppm[80]
Manganese	:	2-68 ppm

Govindarajan and Gopala Rao[81] determined that the vegetative yield was increased by Boron, Zinc, Molybdenum and Vanadium in the soil. Giri et.al.[82]. found that the total mineral contents and calcium decreased after germination in seeds but the Iron content increased.

Other important constituents found in the Dolichos biflorus are, strepogenin[83], β-sitosterol[84], Bulbiformin[85], Linoleic acid[86] (in the seeds oil-30-60%), Polyphenols[87], Oxalates[88] (40% of which was soluble) and Crude fibre(5.3%)[89]

A number of isoflavones have been isolated from the leaves and stems namely Genistein, 2'-hydroxy genistein, dalbergioidin, Kievitone, phaseollidin and isoferrerin (a new compound) after innoculation by some nonpathogenic bacteria, alone with coumestrol and psoralidin by Keen et.al.[90] 2 minor isoflavonoids Dolichin A & B were isolated from the bacteria treated leaves by Ingham et.al.[91] Mitra et.al.[92] isolated another new isoflavone-neohesperidoside. Ciulei et.al.[23]. found a flavone-rutoside and saponins from the seeds.

El-Faki[93] *et.al.* detected 3.6% free sugars-mainly Galactose, Glucose, Sucrose, Raffinose, Stachyose, and verbascose. A low molecular fraction of the water extract (useful as antilithiatic) was recently found to contain mainly-glycerc Mannitol, Galactitol, Glucose, Fructose, Sucrose and m-inositol by Mosin zaman *et.al.*[94].

USES OF DOLICHOS BIFLORUS LINN

The seeds have been used in the indigenous syste medicine for a long time. The Indian Materia Medica lists the traditional uses as:

Actions : Astringent, Diuretic, Tonic.

As galactogue : Decoction of seed powder with unripe *Aegle marmelos and Amaranthus spinosus.* Boiled whole seeds for horses and cows. Plants during flowering as fodder to the milch animals.

In scrofula : Decoction of seed powder with pepper.

In diarrhoea : Expressed juice of plant with catechu

In bowel haemorrhage : Decoction of seeds with cashew nuts.

In leucorrhoea and other menstural derangements : Decoction of seeds.

In Colic : Decoction of seeds with Asafoetida, Ginger powder and Bidalone.

In subacute enlargement of spleen and liver : Soup diet of seeds.

In Piles : Soup diet of seeds.

In cold sweats : Seed powder dusting on skin.

In Bladder and Kidney stones[95] : Decoction of seeds.

In hypertension[95] : Infusion of whole seeds.

Gostowskil *et.al.*[96]. patented an aqueous extract effective in dissolving phosphate type calculi in rats with no toxic side effects. Ground seeds were extracted for 3 hours with Methanol water mixture (1:1) by boiling. It was kept for 15 hrs and evaporated at reduced pressure at a temperature between 50°-60°C. The residue was acidified with phosphoric acid and heated for an hour at 80°C. It is cooled, filtered and extracted with chloroform, The aqueous layer is separated and nutralized with

NaOH. The aqueous extract contained sugars, organic acids, inorganic salts and other polar constituents.

Later Ciulei and coworkers[23] determined the antilithiasis activity of the aqueous extract-in vitro, on human renal calculi on simulated conditions, and obtained 30% disintegration.

Devi and Kurup[97] obtained cholesterol lowering effects in rats by oral administration of seed decoction. Later it was found that the globulin fraction of the extract was responsible for the hypolipidaemic action on rats[98], the insoluble polysaccharides were non effective.

The lectins from the seeds and other parts of *Dolichos biflorus* have many important clinical and immuno histopathological applications. It's use was suggested in legalmedical practice to differentiate human blood from the animal ones[99]. Blood groups A_1 & A_2 determination by the lectin was perfected by Potapov[100]. ABO grouping of human hair using ^{131}I labelled lectinous extract was developed by Boettcher et.al.[101] Oikawa[102] et.al. found that the lectin inhibited in virto fertilization of hamster by cross linkage binding at zona pellucida, and Aubrey et.al.[103] found its inhibitory effect on chick embryonic development. Zalewski and others[104] found that the seed lectin is bound to only C lymphocytes and not T lymphocytes - however it is totally bound to the b cells in chronic lymphocytic lukaemiaindicating its use as a labelling reagent. Kim and Kim[105] suggested the use of lectin as a tracer to differentiate the alveolar cells and cells of lobular carcinoma in breast cancer. Zhang and coworkers[106] determined that the lectin bound to the epithelial cells of only the gastrointestinal and the respiratory tract. Plendl and Schmhal[107] used the lectin for evaluating early lesion patterns in CNS studies. Recently Morgan and coworkers[108] developed a method for improving elicitation of IgG class monoclonal antibodies to tumor-associated antigens and glycoproteins using the *D. biflorus* lectin.

The seeds are also used as horse fodder (which is why the same-horsegram) and as pulses and porridge for human consumption in many tropical countries—including south India. The vegetative part is also used as a fodder and as a green manure due to high mineral composition. Recently Chandrashekhar and coworkers[109] have suggested malted horse gram meal as an inexpensive but nutritious weaning food.

TISSUE CULTURE WORK ON GENUS DOLICHOS

A substantial amount of tissue culture work has been reported on *Dolichos lablab* or the flat bean ('Sem' in Hindi). In 1953, Misra and Samantarai[110] reported induction of rooting in the isolated leaves by treatment with 3 - indolebutyric acid and I-Naphthalene Acetic Acid. Tung and Raghavan[111] in 1968 reported excised root culture studies. Kumar *et.al.*[112]. studied chlorophyll formation and growth of the mesopyll tissue culture by addition of various vitamins and plant growth regulators. It was found that Thiamine, Nicotinic acid, calcium pantothenate, Choline and Inositol induced growth and chlorophyll formation. Kinetin induced growth and chlorophyll formation - which was enhanced by NAA, IAA and Gibberellic acid but inhibited by 2,4-D. Gnanam and Padmanabham[113] studied mesophyll cell suspension culture where 0.02 mg/lt of 2.4-D sustained cell growth without induction of callus. Kumar[114] developed cotyledon callus culture on casein hydrolysate-2,4-D-Kinetin medium and maintained it on Tobacco-highsalt and Murashige and Skoog media to study the role of Ferrous salts on chlorophyll formation. Kulandaivelu and Gnanam[115] cultured isolated leaf cells to study the effects of different plant growth regulators on photosynthetic CO_2 fixation. Optimum physical parameters for mesophyll callus growth were determined by Kumar[116] at ph-5.8, temperature-28°C and light intensity 6000 to 8000 lux. Mohamed and Gnanam[117] found that the isolated leaf cell culture photosynthesize amino acids at the expense of sugars, when incubated with 1 m Mole NH_4OH solution. Choudhuri and Sen[118] found that in the isolated cell cultures Kinetin stimulated DNA, RNA and Protein synthesis, whereas c AMP checked loss of protein with aging.

Dolichos lablab has been shown to biosynthesize many plant growth regulators in high quantities. Yokota and coworkers isolated 3-0-b-D- glucopyranosyl-gibberellin A_1[119] and later (-) Jasmonic acid[120] which was shown to be a new type of plant growth regulator. Later they isolated cytokinins related to zeatin from immature seeds[121].

Tissue culture work on Dolichos biflorus was first reported in 1985 by James, Ghosh and Etzler[122]. They developed callus culture from isolated epicotyl leaves, hypocotyl and roots of germinating seedlings on Murashige and Skoog medium-slightly modified with a higher concentration of Thiamine, Nicotinic acid, Pyridoxine and m-inositol, under continuous fluorecent light and at a temperature of 28°C. The plant growth regulator combinations showing better callus initiation and maintainance were:

(i) 2 ppm 2,4-D + 0.1 ppm Kinetin

(ii) 10.8 ppm 2,4-D = 1 ppm Kinetin

The developed callus was radioammunoassayed for detection of the seed lectin and the cross reactive material (CRM) to the seed lectin found in the stems and leaves. Seed lectin was absent in the callus but the CRM was produced in the callus. However, the above mentioned media with growth regulators did not support CRM formation and the hormone free medium was shown to be the best for this purpose. Sub cellular localization of the CRM was done by immuno fluorescence studies on the sections of the callus.

In 1986, Sinha and Das[123], reported callus development and regeneration of plantlets, from the leaf and anther explants.

In 1988, Spadoro-Tank and Etzler[124] developed cell suspension culture of the stem and cotyledon tissues, which was studied for appearance of the CRM and the related glycoproteins by radioimmunoassay. It was found that the culture synthesized both the seed and the stem/leaf Pectin or CRM. Synthesis was found to be greatly enhanced by heat shock. At 42°C ten time more Petin was produced than at 27°C.

In 1989 Sounder Raj and coworkers[125] reported regeneration of plantlets from the callus grown from the shoot tips by NAA and 6-benzylamiro-purine, which they suggested to be a effective technique for micropropagation of virus free clones.

References

1. Nadkarni, K.M., Indian Materia Medica, pp 458

2. Chopra, R.N., Nayar, S.L. and Chopra, I.C., Glossary of Indian Medicinal Plants, CSIR, New Delhi, pp. 100, (1956)

3. Huang, H., Haung, N. and Li, S., Yaoxue Tongbao, 17(2), 122, (1982)

4. Haung, H., Cheng, C., Lin, W., Yang, G., Song, J., and Ren, G., Zhongguo Yaoli Xuebao, 3(4), 286-8, (1982)

5. Prudhomme, R., Bull. Agr. Intelligence, 13, 494-5, (1923)

6. Fosse, R., Brunel, A., and Thomas, D.E., Compt. rend., 193, 7-11, (1931)

7. Oliver, D., Flora of Tropical Africa, L. Reeve and Co., London, (1971)

8. Vetter, O., Acta. Biol. Med. Ger., 15(1-2), 131-7, (1965)

9. Dardenne, G.A. and Thonart, P., Phytochemistry, 12(2), 473, (1973)

10. Dardenne, G.A., Thonart, P., Otoul, E. and Marschal, R., Phytochemistry, 12(8), 1983-92, (1973)

11. Gunzinger, J., Msonthi, J.D. and Hostettmann, K., Helv. Chim. Acta, 71(1), 72-6, (1988)

12. Martson, A., Gafner, F., Dossji. S.F. and Hostettmann, K, Phytochemistry, 27(5), 1325-6, (1988)

13. Anonymous, Dictionary of Economic Products, Volume III, pp. 175.

14. Anonymous, Flora of British India, Volume II, pp 210

15. Chattopadhyay, N.C., Bnerjee, J., Tah, J.P. and Chakraborty A., Indian Biot., 19(2), 39-43, (1987)

16. Kulkarni, R.N. and Shivashankar, G., Indian J. Exp. 16(3), 404-5, (1978)

17. Anonymous, Wealth of India, Vol. III, Natural Products, CSIR, New Delhi, pp 101., (1986)

18. Mateer, J.G. and Marshall, E.K. (Jr.), J. Biol Chem., 25, 297, (1916)

19. Menon, V.K.N. and Rao, D.N., Indian J. Med. Res., 19(4), 1077, (1952)

20. Venkatasubban, A., Karnal, R., and Dastur N.N., Proc. Indian Acad. Sci., 4B., 370-5, (1936)

21. Damodaran, M., Ramaswamy, R., Venkatesan, T.R., Mahadevan, S. and Ramdas, K., Proc. Indian Acad. Sci., 23B, 86-99, (1946)

22. Damodaran, M. and Venkatesan, T.R., Proc. Indian Acad. Sci., 27B, 26-32, (1948)

23. Ciulei, I., Istudor, V., Mihele, D., Joja., I. and Apostol, E., Farmacia, 32(3), 129-35, (1984)

24. Narayana, N., J. Indian Instt. Sci., 13A, 153-8, (1930)

25. Rao, M.R.R. and Sreenivasaya, M., Curr. Sci., 15,25-6, (1946)

26. Bagchi, S.P. Ganguli, N.C. and Roy, S.C., Ann Biochem. Expt' Med., 15, 149-54, (1955)

27. Radhakrishnan, A.N., Vaidyanathan, C.S. and Giri, K.V., J. Indian Instt. Sci., 37A, 178-94, (1955)

28. Palacios, G. and Bari, A., Proc. Indian Acad. Sci., 3B, 334-61, (1936)

29. Rajagopalan, N., Curr. Sci., 33(15), 454-6, (1964)

30. Kuznetsova, A.A., Murdov, K.M., and Kazautseva, V.N., Izv. Akad. Nauk. Turkm, SSR, Ser. Biol, Nauk., 5, 19-23 (1975)

31. Sudhakar, C., Reddy, P.S. and Veeranjaneyulu, K., Indian J. Exp. Biol., 25(7), 479-82, (1987).

32. Sudhakar, C. and Veeranjaneyulu,K., Indian J. Exp. Biol, 26(8), 618-20, (1988)

33. Niyogi, S.P. Narayana, N. and Desai, B.G., Indian J. Med. Res. 19. 175-83, (1931)

34. Ray, P.K., Indian J. Nutr. Diet, 7(1), 1-4, (1970).

35. Pant, R., Nair, C.R. and Singh, K.S., Curr. Sci., 37(6), 166-7, (1968).

36. Manage, L. and Sohonie, K., J. Food Sci. Technol., 9(1), 35-6, (1972)

37. Abdi, H. and Sahile, M.K., J. Food Sci Technol., 13(5), 237-9, (1976)

38. Sayanova, V.V. and Sumenkova, V.V. Izv. Akad. Nauk. Mold. SSR. Ser. Biol. Khim, Nauk., 5, 23-8, (1977)

39. Begum, J.M., Srihara, P. and Hiremath, S.R., Mysore J. Agric. Sci., 11(4), 521-4, (1977).

40. Singh, G. and Bird, G.W.G., J. Sci. Ind. Res. 15C, 182-3, (1956)

41. Bird. G.W.G., Vox Sang., 4, 307-13, (1959)

42. Ensgraber, A., Kruepe, M. and Eusgraber-Hattingen, R., Z. Immunitactsforsch., 120, 340-66, (1960)

43. Gray; M.F., VS : 3053379, (1962)

44. Kuehnemund, O., Kochler, W. and Prokop, O., Hoppe-Seylers Z. Physiol. Chem., 349(10), 1434-6, (1968)

45. Etzler, M.E. and Kabat, E.A., Biochemistry, 9(4), 869-77, (1970)

46. Font. J., Leseney, A.M. and Bourrillon, R., Biochim. Biophys, Acta. 243(3), 343-46, (1971)

47. Manage, L., Joshi, A. and Sohonie, K., Toxicon, 10(1), 89-91, (1972)

48. Pere, M., Font, J. and Bourrillon, R., Biochim, Biophys. Acta, 365(1), 40-6, (1974)
49. Carter, W.G., Diss, Abstr. Int. B, 35(10), 4794, (1975)
50. Carter, W.G., and Etzler, M.E., Biochemistry, 14(23), 5118-22, (1975)
51. Etzler, M.E., Talbot, C.F. and Ziaya, P.R., FEBS Lett., 82(1), 39-4, (1977)
52. Carter, W.G. and Sharon, N, Arch. Biochem. Biophys., 180(2), 150-82, (1977).
53. Talbot, C.F. and Etzler, M.E., Biochemistry, 17(8), 1474-9, (1978)
54. Talbot, C.F., Diss. Abstr. Int.B., 41(5), 1756, (1980)
55. Talbot, C.F., and Etzler, M.E., Plant Physiol., 61(5), 847-50, (1978)
56. Lorentz, K., Flatler, B and Kolle, F.W., J. Clin. Chem. Clin. Biochem., 17(11), 757-65, (1979)
57. Etzler, M.E., Phytopathology, 71(7), 744-6, (1981)
58. Etzler, M.E., J. Biosci., 5 (Suppl.-1), 1-7, (1983)
59. Handa, G., Singh, J., Nandi, L.N., Sharma, M.L. and Atal, C.K., Indian Drugs, 23(5), 264-8, (1986)
60. Quinn, J.M., Diss. Abstr. Int. B. 48(3), 745, (1988)
61. Schnell, D.J. and Etzler, M.E., J. Biol. Chem., 263(29), 648-53, (1988)
62. Schnell, D.J., Diss. Abstr. Int. B, 49(4), 1156, (1988)
63. Quinn, J.M. and Etzler, M.E., Plant Physiol., 91(4), 1382-6, (1989)
64. Bhimeshwar, B. and Sreenivasaya, N., J. Sci. Ind. Res (India), 9B(1), 23-4, (1950)
65. Mukunden, M.A., Sundaram, T.K. Shanmugasundaram E.R.B., Curr. Sci., 30, 461-2, (1961)
66. Meyer, D. and Bourillon, R., Biochimie, 55(1), 5-10, (197)
67. Mary, A., and Sastry, K.S., Phytochemistry, 17(3), 397-9, (1978)
68. Mehta, S.L. and Simlot, M.H., J. Biosci., 4(3), 295-306, (1982)
69. Sudhakar, C., Reddy, P.S. and Veeranjaneyulu K., Indian J. Exp. Biol., 25(7), 479-82, (1987)
70. Makhijani, J.K., and Bannerjee B.N., Indian J. Vet. Sci Animal Husbandry, 8, 13-28, (1938).

71. Sohonie, K. and Misra, V.C., Brit. J. Nutr., 4, 134-8, (1950)

72. Dakshinamurti, K., Curr. Sci., 24, 194-5, (1955)

73. Chitre, R.G., Desai, D.B. and Raut, V.S. Indian J. Med. Res., 43, 575-83, (1955)

74. Iengar, N.G.C., Jayaram, V. and Rau, Y.V.S., Ann. Biochem, Exptt. Med., 15, 39-45, (1955)

75. Raut, V.S. and Chitre, R.G., J. Postgrad. Med., 7, 35-7, (1961)

76. Sastry, K.S.K. and Appaiah, K.M., Mysore J. Agr. Sci., 2(2), 106-10, (1968)

77. Nazir, D.J. and Magar, N.G., Indian J. Chem., 1, 278-9, (1963)

78. Pore, M.S., Indian J. Agric. Sci., 49(9), 712-14, (1979)

79. Pore, M.S., ibid, 49(7), 532-4, (1979)

80. Yousuf, M. and Venkatachalam, G., Indian Vet. J., 55(11), 924-5, (1978)

81. Govindarajan, S.V. and Gopalarao, H.G., J. Indian Soc. Soil Sci., 12, 355-61, (1964)

82. Giri, J., Parvatham, R. and Santhini, K., Indian J. Nutr. Diet, 18(3), 87-91, (1981)

83. Krishnamurthy, K. and De, S.S., Indian J. Physiol. Allied Sci., 5, 83-9, (1951)

84. Chakraborty, R.J., Chakraborty, D., Mitra, M.N., Dasgupta B. and Maiti, P.C., Indian J. Ind. Res., 15C, 89-90, (1956)

85. Vasudeva, R.S., Singh, P., Sengupta, P.K., Mahmood, M. and Bajaj, B.S., Ann. Appl. Biol., 51(3), 415-23, (1963)

86. Mahadevappa, V.G. and Raina, P.L., J. Agric Food Chem., 26(5), 1241-3, (1978)

87. Satwadhar, P.N., Kadam, S.S. and Salunkhe, D.K., Qual. Plant-Plant Foods Hum. Nutr., 31(1), 71-6, (1981)

88. Meena, B.A., Umapathy, K.P., Pankaja, N. and Prakash, J., J. Food Sci. Technol., 24(1), 43-4, (1987).

89. Kumary, M.N.P., Fathima, A. and Saraswathi, G., J. Food Sci. Technol., 21(2), 95-7, (1984)

90. Keen, N.T. and Ingham, J.L., Z Naturforsch., C:Biosci., 35C(11-12), 923-6, (1980)

91. Ingham, J.L., Keen, N.T., Markham, K.R. and Mulheim, L.J., Phytochemistry, 20(4), 807-9, (1981).

92. Mitra, J., Das, A. and Joshi, T., Phytochemistry, 22(4), 1063-4, (1985)

93. El-Faki, H.A., Desikachar, H.S.R., Paramahans, S and Tharanathan, R.N., Starch, 35(5), 163-6 (1983)

94. Mosinuzzaman, M., Islam, M.S. and Nahar, N., Dhaka Univ. Stud. Part B, 37(1), 11-17, (1989)

95. Bhattacharya, K., Drvyagguna Sahgraha, 4th ed., P. Prakashan, Calcutta, pp. 401-50, (1952)

96. Gustowskii, W., Kocor, M., Atal, C.K., Orkiszewski A., Olozewskii, R. and Wrocinskii, T., POo. PL 11532:5, (1982)

97. Devi, K.S. and Kurup, P.A. Atherosclerosis, 11(3) 479-84, (1970)

98. Prema, L. and Kurup, P.A., Atherosclerosis, 18(3) 369-77, (1973)

99. Mackerle, S., Acta Univ. Palacki. Olomuc. Fac. Med., 38, 199-228, (1965)

100. Potapov, M.I., Probl. Gematol. Pereliv. Krovi, 12(3), 13-16, (1967)

101. Boettcher, B. and Kay, D.J., Vox. Sang., 25(5), 420-5, (1973)

102. Oikawa, T., Nicholson, G.L. and Yanagimachi, R., Exp. Cell Res., 83(2), 239-46, (1974)

103. Aubrey, M. and Bourillon, R., IRCS Libr. Compend., 1(7), 1.2.7. (1973)

104. Zalewski, P.D., Forbes, I.J., Khlenbriick, G. and Valente L. Clin. Exp. Immunol., 44(2), 304-14, (1981)

105. Kim, C.S. and Kim, S.M., Koryo Tachakkyo Uikwa Tachak Nonmuniji, 22(1), 375-83, (1985)

106. Zhang, K., Shi, D., Fu x. and Liu, S., Xhonghua Yixue Zazhi, 65(3), 144-7, (1985).

107. Plendl, J. and Schmahl, W., Comm. Eur. Communities, (Rep.) EVR, EVR-10414, Radiat, Risks Dev. Nerce, Syot., 61-72, (1986)

108. Morgan, A.C.(Jr.), McIntyre, R., Woodhouse, C.S. and Abrams, P.G., U.S.-US4822734 (11.435-68, C12 P12/00), (1989)

109. Chandrashekhar, U., Bhooma, N. and Reddy, S., Indian. Nutr. Diet, 25(2), 37-43, (1988)

110. Misra, G. and Samantarai, B., J. Indian Bot. Soc, **32**, 127-30, (1953)

111. Tung. H.F. and Raghavan, V., Ann. Bot., 32(127), 509-19, (1968)

112. Kumar, A., Kant, V. and Arya, H.C., Indian J. Exp. Biol., 10 (1), 65-7, (1972)

113. Gnanam, A. and Padmanabhan, D., Curr. Sci., 43(17), 559-60, (1974)

114. Kumar, A., Indian J. Exp. Biol., 12(6), 595-6, (1974).

115. Kulandaivelu, G. and Gnanam, A., Physiol. Plant, 33(3), 234-40, (1975)

116. Kumar, A., Phytomorphology, 24(1-2), 96-101, (1974)

117. Mohamed, A.H. and Gnanam A., Plant Biochem. J. 4(1), 1-9, (1977)

118. Chaoudhuri, C. and Sen, S.P., Plant Biochem. J., 7(1), 37-53, (1980)

119. Yokote, T., Kobayashi, S., Yamane, H. and Takahashi, N., Agric. Biol. Chem., 42(9), 1811-12, (1978)

120. Yamane, H., Takagi, H., Abe, H., Yokote, T. and Takahashi, N., Plant Cell Physiol., 22(4), 689-97, (1981)

121. Yokota, T., Ueda, J. and Takahashi, N., Phytochemistry, 20(4), 683-6, (1981)

122. James, D.W., Ghosh, M. and Etzler, M.E., Plant Physiol., 77(3), 630 4, (1985)

123. Sinha, R.R. and Das, K., Curr. Sci., 55, 447, (1986)

124. Spadoro-Tank, J.P. and Etzler, M.E., Plant Physiol., 88(4), 1131-5, (1988)

125. Sounder Raj, V., Tejavathi, D.H. and Nijalingappa, B.H.M., Curr. Sci., 58(24), 1385-8, (1989)

7

Ipomoea hederacea Auct; Non Jacq

Ipomoea Linn (Convolvulaceae)

A large genus of twining, creeping floating or erect herbs, rarely shrubs or trees, widely distributed throughout the tropical and warm temperate region of the world. About 50 species are found in India, the most important being *I.batatas* (sweet potato) extensively cultivated for its edible root tubers. A number of species have been introduced into India and many species are grown in gardens for ornamental purposes, some are of medicinal value. The following species of Ipomoea are used medicinally[1].

1. *Ipomoea hederacea*
2. *I. purpurea*
3. *I. pestigridis*
4. *I. aquatica*
5. *I. carnosa*
6. *I. fistulosa*
7. *I pes-caprae*
8. *I. murocoides*
9. *I. cadaefoli*
10. *I. decasperma*
11. *I. reptans*
12. *I. violaceae*
13. *I. quamoclit*
14. *I. muricata*
15. *I. eriocapra*
16. *I. maxima*
17. *I. obscura*
18. *I. uniflora*

A number of species of lpomoea other than those mentioned are of minor importance, either as ornamental plants or medicinal plants. They are:-

19. *I. angulata* lan, syn. *I. coccinea* non Linn.,
20. *I. Phonenicea* Roxb
21. *Quamoclit phoeniceae* Choisy
22. *I. Coptica* (Linn) Roth syn *I. dissecta* Willd
23. *I. Dasysperma* Jacq
24. *I. Dichroa* Choisy syn. *I. pilosa*
25. *I. Ficifolia* Lindl.
26. *I. Gracilis* R. Br.
27. *I. Illustris* Prain syn. *I. campanulata* auct., non Linn
28. *I. Campanulata* Linn
29. *I. learii* Paxt
30. *I. Tilliacea* (Willd) Choisy syn. *I. fastigiata* (Roxb).

Several other species are grown in Indian gardens exclusively for their showy flowers. They include,

31. *I. Hederacea* Linn Syn. *Convulvulus hederaceus* (Linn)
32. *I. Hors falliae* Hook
33. *I. Lobata* (Ceru.) syn. *I. versicolour* Meissn.
34. *I. Macrorhiza* Mich.
35. *I. Tricolor* Cav. syn. *I. rubrocaerulea* Hook.

MORPHOLOGY OF IPOMCEA HEDERACEA

Ipomoea hederacea (auct,: non Jacq)
Synonym : Ipomoea nill (Linn) Roth 2, 3
Regional Names :

Sanskrit	-	Krishnablija, Shyamabija.
Hindi	-	Kaladana, mirchai,
Beng	-	Kaladanah, nilkalmi,
Mar	-	Nilpushpi, nilyel
Guj	-	Kaladana, Kal kumpan,
Tel	-	Jirika, Kolli.
Tam	-	Kakkattan, sirikki.
Kan	-	Ganribija,
Oriya	-	Khanaikhondo.
Deccan	-	Kalizirki., zirki.
Kashmir	-	Hub-ul-nil.
Punjab	-	Bildi, ishpecha, ker, kirpawa, phaprusag.

Unani Tibbi - Iurtum Hindi, Tukhm-e-Nilopaich, Ishq-paicha, Kubku.

English - Pharbitis Seeds.

Habitat : An extensive, hairy, herbaceous annual or perennial twiner, found throughout India upto a height of 6,000 feet in the Himalayas; it is frequently grown in gardens for its ornamental flowers, and often runs wild in hedges and waste places.

Period of Occurrence - Flowers and fruits occur from August to October

Description : A spreading herbaceous twiner; stems retorsely hairy; leaves ovate-cordate; 3 - lobed; flowers in axillary stout peduncled; 1-2 flowered reduced cymes; deep blue tinged with pink; bracts linear; calyx 5, slightly connate at base, obtuse, upto 2 cm.long, hairy at base and on margins; corolla funnel shaped, tube constricted at mouth, narrow; stamens 5, filaments hairy at base, style long, stout at base, slender; stigma lanceolate; fruit a capsule, 3 - celled, 6 - ovuled sub-globose, dull brown glabrous, seeds glabrous.

Parts used : seeds. The dried seeds of I. hederacea are sold in bazaars under the name of KALADANA and used as purgative. The seeds are black in colour except for a brownish spot at the hilum, small in size (1/4-1/3 inch in length), angular and of the shape of the segment of a sphere, 100 seeds weigh 3-4g. Taste at first sweetish, later acrid and disagreeable.

Procedure and *time of collection* : Air dried capsules are collected.

Preservation and *storage* : Air dried seeds (under shade) should be stored in dry and cold place and can be preserved for three years.

Use : Kaladana is an active cathartic and is official in the Indian Pharmacopoeia. It is used as a substitute for *jalap* (*Exogonium purga* Benth). The purgative action is due to a resin which is extracted from the seeds along with inert resinous matter by alcohol. Both seeds and the total resin extract are employed as cathartic in doses of 30-45 gr. and 4-8gr, respectively. In overdoses they produce symptoms of irritant poisoning. Other preparations of Kaladana used in medicine include an extract, a tincture and a compound powder (Pulvis Kaladanae compositus) consisting of seeds, potassium hydrogen tartrate and powdered ginger[4,5,6].

PHYTOCHEMICAL WORK ON IPOMOMEA HEDERACEA

A review of the research work reported on *Ipomoea hederacea* auct, non Jacq, indicates that this plant has mainly been evaluated for the phytochemical studies. A number of workers reported studies on the chemical examination of seeds of *Ipomoea headeracea.*

The chemical composition of *Ipomoea hederacea* is as follows[7,8,9,10,11].

Constitutes : Commercial samples of Kaladana contain 14-15% of crude resinous matter with nauseating acrid taste and disagreeable odour: the resin can be fractionated into a glycosidal part and a non-glycosidal part. The activity of the drug was formerly attributed to the glycosidal fraction, namely pharbitsin, consisting, of an ether soluble portion (tiglic acid, methy-ethyl acetic acid, and α-methyl-β orybutric acid) an ether - insoluble portion (pharbitinic acid), giving on hydrolysis glucose, *rhamnose* and ipurolic acid. More recent work has shown that the glycosidal resin is inert: the activity of the drug resides in the non-glycosidal resin (2% of the drug) and causes copious purgation in doses of 250 mg.

Besides the resinous matter, the seeds contain a fixed oil (12.4%) and small mounts of saponin, mucilage and tannin. Extracted oil pale yellow in colour with an unpleasant odour and has the following characteristics:

Sp. gravity	: 0.918
Sap value	: 190.48
Acetyl value	: 5.19
Acid value	: 3.45
Iod. value	: 121.5
Unsapon.matter	: 1.98%
Mixed fatty acids contained	
Palmitic	: 5.93%
Stearic	: 20.37%
Arachidic	: 7.79%
Behenic	: 1.29%
Linolenic	: 5.99%
Linoleic	: 14.54%
Oleic	: 43.98%

The unsaponifiable matter contains coprosterol[12,13]. The flowers contain anthocyanin pigments. The colouring matter of red flowers is pelargonin chloride. Deep violet and red violet flowers contain peonin chloride[14].

Khanna *et. al.*[15] have established standards for seeds of *I. hederacea* as given in the following table.

DATA RELATING TO STANDARDS FOR SEEDS OF *I. HEDERACEA*

Table 7.1

Sample	Wt.in.g of 100 Seeds	Ash %	Lod %	% Extractive Solubleun		
				Alcohol	Water	Pet.ether
1.	5.6	4.46	8.9	13.2	24.5	10.00
2.	5.8	4.9	7.7	14.0	29.7	11.5
3.	6.0	4.25	8.1	12.9	29.0	10.7
4.	5.6	4.53	9.7	14.1	29	10.6

Each result was the average of 4 experiments

Marderosian *et. al.*[16] have reported the results of indole alkaloid determination of seeds of twenty nine different species and varieties of *Ipomoea*. A modification of the procedure of Hofmann used. Seeds of *Ipomoea headeracea* from different sources did not shown any presence of indole alkaloids.

Investigations on indole base of *I. hederacea* were carried out by Prakash M.S.[17] *et. al.* Estimation of total indole bases in 2 different samples of seeds revealed content as 0.0058 and 0.055% on dry wt. basis. The chloroform extract of seeds giving the higher content of bases on subjecting to 2-D T.L.C. revealed the presence of fifteen Ehrlich positive spots. Detailed chromatographic studies and other chromatographic work showed of the bases identical with isolysergol.

TISSUE CULTURE WORK ON GENUS IPOMOEA

A review of the research work reported on tissue culture of genus Ipomoea revealed that only a few species of Ipomoea have been evaluated through tissue culture for the study of their chemical constituents. The tissue culture studies have been mainly taken for *Ipomoea batatas, Ipomoea violaceae* (Morning glory), Ipomoea nil (L) Roth (Pharbitis Nill chois, Japanese Morning glory[18].

The first successful attempt to develop and examine morning glory tissue cultures was done by Staba and Laursen in 1966[19]. They examined three varieties of *I. violaceae* L. cv flying saucer (FS), cv heavenly blue (HB) and cv pearly gates (PG) seed callus tissue cultures for indole alkaloids by thin layer chromatography and spectrophotometry. In addition the seeds of plants of these three varieties, the seeds of three varieties of Japanese morning glory cv matzukaze, yuki and chiyono okina,were also examined. These workers showed that the seeds and aerial portions of three *Ipomoea violaceae*. While traces of indole alkaloids were contained in the roots callus tissue, and callus medium for these varieties and the seeds of three Japanese morning glory varieties. They showed the absence of alkaloids in the Heavenly blue tissue cultures but they could detect that although callus tissue cultures more consistently contained in the root callus tissue, and callus medium for these varieties and the seeds of three Japanese morning glory varieties. They showed the absence of alkaloids in the heavenly blue tissue cultures but they could detect that although callus tissue cultures more constantly contained alkaloids than their respective medium, the medium extract occasionally was found to give a more positive and complex pattern than the callus extract on thin layer plates.

This work was forwarded to progress when Dobberstein and Staba[21] examined the suspension cultures of *Ipomoea violaceae* var. pearly gates in medium containing various chemical factors that might stimulate indole alkaloid production.

Although seeds of *Ipomoea violaceae* var. pearly gates were reported to contain from 0.015 to 0.02% total alkaloids[16] however these authors reported lower percentage of alkaloids. Through their investigation *Ipomoea violaceae* var. pearly gates callus and media were found to contain 0.92 mg/p 100 gms wet weight total alkaloids.

A further investigation with the major objective of studying the metabolic rates for major nutrients in suspension cultures of Ipomoea species (morning glory) was undertaken by Rose et. al.[22].

Song and Tattrie studied the lipid composition of morning glory cells grown in suspension cultures and determined the total fatty acids of morning glory (*Ipomoea* species) cells grown in suspension cultures for 8 days[23]. Veliky established the effect of pH on tryptophol formation by cultured plant cells of *Ipomoea* species by growing cultures of Ipomoea species in a chemically defined medium containing DL-tryptophan[14]. One of the metobolites was identified as tryptophol and its formation was studied under various growth conditions. It was reported that in the normal uncontrolled formentations tryptophol concentration reached a maximum level of 9mg/litre in 48 hours. It was also shown that in the formentation controlled at PH 6.3 tryptophol formation was stimulated by 71% measured at the peak of its concentration in medium, 96 hours after inoculation, however, controlling the pH at 4.8 resulted in an inhibition of tryptophol formation.

Another important species, evaluated through tissue culture for its chemical constituents is *Ipomoea batatas* (sweet potato). Biosynthesis of furanoterpenes by sweet potato cell culture was reported by Oba and Uritani, where callus was induced from sweet potato root tissue on agar medium containing Heller's vitamins, 2, 4-D, yeast extract and sucrose[25].

References

1. Kirtikar, K.R., Basu B.D., in Indian Medicinal Plants vol. III (2nd Ed), 1711-1714
2. Flora of British India, IV, 199.
3. Ahuja A., Verma M., Grewal S., Ind. J. Exp. Biol. 1982, **20**, 455.
4. Flora of Malesiana, Ser, I, **4**(4), 465.
5. Bentley and Trimen, III, 185.
6. Indian Pharmacopiea, 1966, 354, 509.
7. British Pharmaceutical Codex, 1949, 459.
8. Sen Gupta and Gupta. K. *Indian. J. Pharm*, 1948, **10**, 106.
9. Wehme II, 1012.
10. U.S.D., 1955, 1728.
11. B.P.C. 1949, 460.
12. Chemical Abstracts, 1924, **18**, 1879.
13. Kathpalia and Dutt. *Ind. Soap. J.* 1947, 48, **13**, 77.
14. Chemical Abstracts, 1927, **21**, 2391.
15. Thakkar and Singh, *Indian Farming* 1953-54, **3**(10), 12.
16. Kauna, L.V. *et. al., Indian J. Pharm*, 1959, **21**, (12), 341.

17. Marderosian Der are and Young Jr., H.W., *Lloydia* 1966, **29**(1), 35-42.
18. Prakash M.S. and Banerjee S.K., *Ind. J. Pharm*, 1976, **38**(6) 157, B25.
19. Nakayama S., Borthwick, H.A., Hendricks., S.B., *Bot Gaz*, 1960, **121**, 237.
20. Staba E.J. and Pant C., J. J. Pharm. Sci., 1966, **55**(10), 1099.
21. Dobberstein, R.H., and Staba E.J., *Lloydia*, 1969, **32**, 141
22. Rose D.S., Martin M., and Clay P.D.F., *Can. J. Bot*, 1972, **50**, 1201.
23. Song M., and Tattrie N., Can. J. Bot., 1973, **51**, 1893
24. Veliky I.A., *Lloydia*, 1977, **40**, 5.
25. Ohja K., and Uritani, *Plant Cell Physiol*, 1979, **20**, 819.

8
Mallotus philippinensis Muell Arg.

Mallotus philippinensis Muell. Arg. (Fig. 8.1) belongs to the family *Euphorbiaceae* and is used medicinally in the Philippine Islands. It is a dioecious shrub or much branched short tree branchlets, young leaves and inflorescence tawny or rusty pubescent. About 20 species are found in India. It is commonly known in *Hindi:* Kamala, Kambila, Rohini, in *English: Monkey face tree, in Bengali:* Kamala, in *Marathi;* Shendri, in *Gujarati:* Kapilo, in *Telegu:* Kunkuma, Sinduri, Chendiramu, in *Tamil:* Kapli Kungumam in *Malayalam:* Kuramadakku, in *Nepal:* Sindure, in *Assam:* Jorat.

DISTRIBUTION

Widely distributed throughout tropical India long the fast of Himalaya from Kashmir eastwards upto 5,000 ft. all over the Punjab, Uttar Pradesh, Bengal, Assam, Burma, Singapore, and from Sind southwards to Bombay and Ceylon. It is also reported as growing in China, the Malaya Islands, Australia, Pakistan and Andaman Islands.

MORPHOLOGY OF LEAVES

Alternate, variable in size 7.5-15 cm., by 3.2-7.5 cm., ovate or oate lanceolate, acuminate, entire or slightly toothed, glabrous above, pubescent and with numerous orbicular red glands beneath reticulately veined, base rounded or acute, strongly 3-nerved at the base and with 4-7 pairs of nerves above the basal ones: petioles 2.5-5 cm. long, cylindric, fulvous pubescent with two small sessile glands one on each side of the summit (Fig.1).

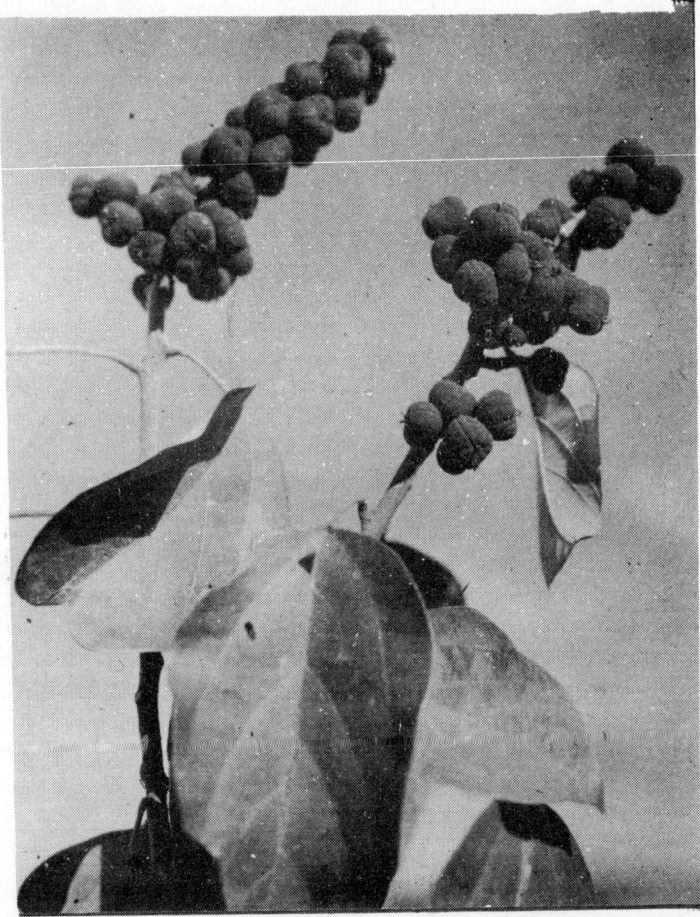

Fig. 8.1 The Fruiting Branch of Mallotus Philippinesis Muell. Arg.

MORPHOLOGY OF FLOWERS

Dioecious, small, the male clustered sessile or very shortly pedicellate, in erect terminal spikes which are usually several together and often longer than the leaves; the female sessile are nearly so, in short spikes.

Male Flowers

Sepals 4 (rarely 5), 3 mm long, lanceolate, acute. Stamens numerous. bracts 15 mm long, broadly ovate, acute. buds-globosely ovoid.

Female Flowers

Calyx divided nearly to the base, sepals 3 or 4, thicker than in the male, ovate-lanceolate.

Ovary with red glands, 3-celled; styles 3 simple papillose, Capsules 8-13 mm in diameter, 3-lobed, loculicidally 3-valved, covered with a bright red powder consisting of minute stelltae hairs and fine grains of a red resinous substance soluble in alcohol and ether.

MORPHOLOGY OF FRUITS

Dehiscent, anther 2 locular. The fruit is 3-valved capsule coloured red from the numerous red glands upon it.

MORPHOLOGY OF SEEDS

4 mm in diameter, subglobose, thick, black in colour and about 7000 maunds can be collected annually in India.

MEDICINAL USES

The crude powder of kamala obtained as a glandular pubescence from the exterior of fruits is found to be anthelminitic in activity and active against thread worm, hook worms and round worm and earth worms. The anthelminitic activity is due to rottlerin and isoallorottlerin. It has been found that rottlerin is toxic but isoallorottlerin exhibits greater activity than rottlerin. A 50: 50 mixture of rottlerin and isoallorottlerin is more active than either of them alone. The pentamethyl ester of rottlerin possess no anthelminitic activity. The drug was found to be 100% effective against tape worms. It was also found that time required to cause death does not vary in proportion to concentration i.e. on doubling the concentration of the drug time required to kill the worm is not halved[1-3].

The granular brick red kamala powder was tried in the form of a liquid extract in doses of 1 to 3 fluid drachm every three hours until three doses were administered. A purgative of castor oil was given thereafter and it was found to be efficacious in expelling round and thread worm[3].

The glands on fruits are bitter pungent, heating, purgative, cathartic, styptic, anthelmintic, vulnerary, detergent, maturant, carminative, heal ulcers and wounds, tumours, stone in the bladder, useful in bronchitis, enlargement of spleen. The hairs and glands are also useful in scabies, ringworm and other skin diseases in Uanni system, lessen intestinal pain and also useful in jaundice and as a constituent of Arshina ointment which is used to cure piles. Oral administration in the form of emulsion reduces fertility in female rats and guineapigs. The effect is however temporary and the animal retrun to normal after the drug is withdrawn[4-7].

Kamala was formely used in India for dyeing silk and wool to a bright orange colour and it is still used for this purpose to a limited extent and for colouring soaps, oils, ice-cream, and drinks. The rottlerin and its pentapotassium derivatives are employed for colouring foodstuffs. lemonades, lime juice and other beverages. It is also used as a sindhur or kumkum by women in India[8,9].

The fruits of the plant are used for making dyes and insect repellents, kernels effective in anthelmintic, rheumatism and snake bite treatment. The red powder on fruits when mixed with some oil is a good remedy for ulcers.[10].

The leaves are bitter, cooling give appetite cause flatulence and constipation[3],

The decoction of bark is used in abdominal pain. it is a nurse plant for sal in the lower hills. Wood is used for making implements.[11].

Among the tribe of Chota Nagpur the root, well ground is rubbed on the painful parts in articular rheumatism.

In katha., Burma, the seeds are ground to a paste and applied to wounds and cuts[3].

The powdered seeds are mixed with sulphur and sandalwood oil and the mixture is very effective when applied externally in rheumatic joints and also in dermatitis. Seeds are also used as a source of dye (1.4-3.7%)[12, 13].

PHYTOCHEMICAL INVESTIGATION ON MALLOTUS PHILIPPINESIS MUELL ARG.

The tree is mainly known for the kamala powder which consists of glandular and stellate non-glandular hairs from the capsules of the plant, and has long been used as an anthelmintic and as an orange dye for silk. According to early chemical investigation, kamala contains phenolic compounds of which rottlerin (mallotoxin) is the main compound. The compound was first isolated by Anderson[14] (1855). As a result of extensive studies by British[15-19]. Indian[20, 21] and German[22, 23] investigators before world war II The structure (Ia) was accepted for rottlerin[18]. Narang et al[20, 21] (1937) also isolated a substance with recorded properties of isoallorotterin (II) (iso-rottlerin) from extracts of kamala. The structure of isoallorottlerin (II) was determined by synthesis by Brockmann and Mater[22] and McGookin et al[19] but its natural occurrence could, however, not be conclusively confirmed, Cardillo et. al.[24] (1965) isolated two additional compounds from kamala, which they called 3-hydroxy rottlerin (Ib) and 3,4 dihydroxyrottlerin (Ic). No isoallorottlerin (II) was found. Crombie et al[25] (1968) isolated two new compounds from kamala extracts, lacking the methylene bridge, which they called "red compound" and "yellow compound". The structures (III) and (IV), respectively, were proposed for these compounds.

R$_1$ = R$_2$ = H: Rottlerin (Ia)
R$_1$= H: R$_2$ = OH: 3-hydroxy rottlerin (Ib)
R$_1$= R$_2$ = OH: 3,4 dihydroxy rottlerin (Ic)

By ether extraction of kamala and column chromatography on silica gel, four phloroglucinol derivaties, namely rottlerin (Ia), isoallorottlerin (II), red compound (III) and "yellow compound" (IV), could be isolated in crystalline form. In addition a further substance methylene-bis-methyl-phloroacetophenone (V) was identified in trace amounts with TLC by comparison with a synthetic sample. The ether extract of kamala also contained, two additional minor compounds, kamalin 1 and kamalin 2, the structure of which had not yet been elucidated.

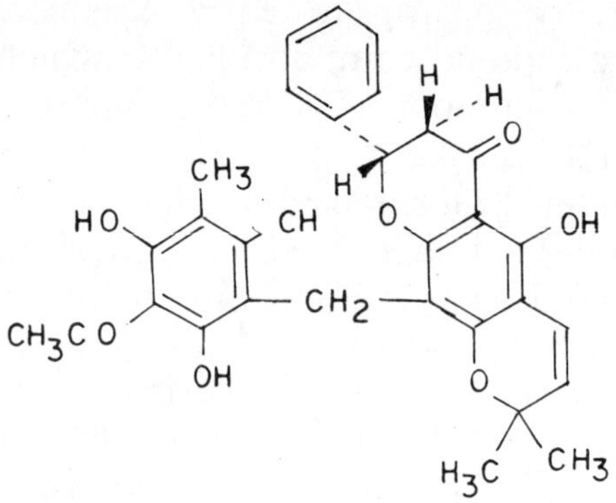

Isoallorottlerin (II)

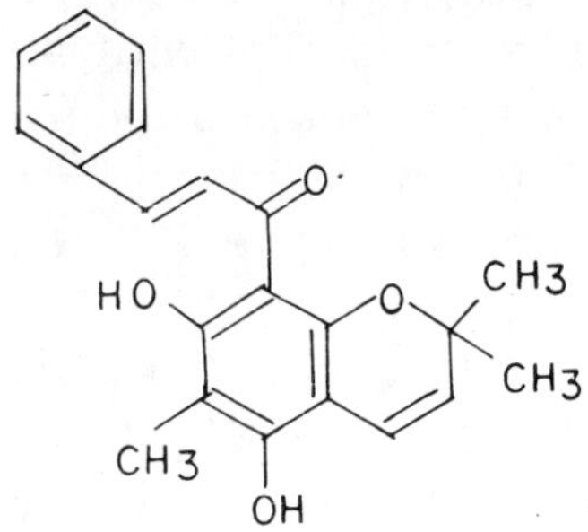

Red compound (III)

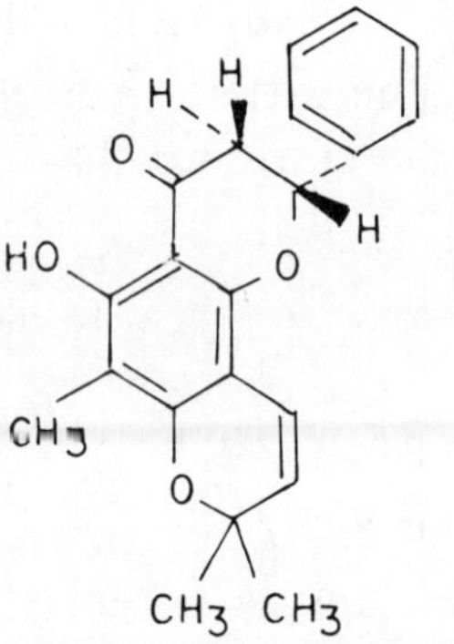

Yellow compound (IV)

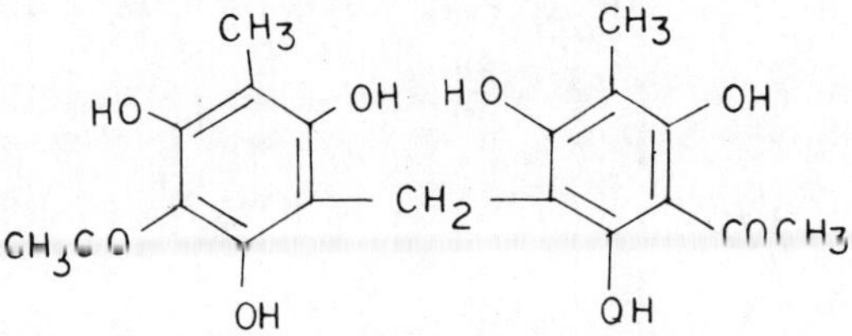

Methylene-bis-methylphloroacetophenone (V)

The absence of 3-hydroxy rottlerin (Ib) and 3,4 dihydroxy rottlerin (Ic) in some samples, could be due to chemical variability of the drug from different geographical sources.

The composition of phloroglucinol derivatives is relatively constant in materials of different origins.

Composition of phloroglucinol derivatives isolated from kamala[26]

Rottlerin (Ia) 60%
Red compound (III) 30%
Yellow compound (IV) 5%
Isoallorottlerin (V) 5%
Methylene-bis-methylphloroacetophenone ....traces

Kamalin 1...traces
Kamalin 2...traces

Kamala also contains other compounds like wax, traces of volatile oils, tannins, sugar, gum, starch, cellulosic materials, oxalic acid, citric acid and mineral matter[27].

Kamala is used as dye by local people. It is harmless and odourless and is very stable. Kamala dye when dissolved in fats in small amount gives a light yellow colour which is natural to butterfat of good quality. The effect of addition of this substance in small concentration on the oxidation of fat was measured by oxygen absorption at 95°C and it was seen that induction period is considerably increased by the addition of even 0.02% of kamala dye. The rate of oxygen absorption is also reduced by the addition of this inhibitor[28].

The leaves of *Mallotus philippinesis* Muell Arg. contains nitrogen and ash. The nitrogen content was estimated by Kjeldahl's method and found to be 2.14% and for the determination of ash content, the leaves were ashed in silica crucible in a muffle furnace at 600-700°C and was found to be 13.37%[29]. Leaves also contain bergenin in very minute amounts.

Petroleum ether extract (60-80°C) of heartwood of tree yielded betulin-3-acetate by chromatography over silica gel as a major compound and the other compounds are lupeol acetate, sitosterol and lupeol and the alcoholic extract yielded bergenin as a major compound.

The bark of the tree contains about 6-10% tannins[30] and the petroleum ether extract on chromatography over silica get yielded acetylaleuritolic acid (0.006%)[31].

Robberts and coworkers[32] (1963) isolated pharmacologically active cardiac glycosides from seeds of *M. phillippinensis*.

The Cardenolides obtained are:

    (I)   Corotoxigenin L-rhamnoside
    (II)   Coroglaucigenin L-rhamnoside

A number of solvents are used for the extraction of kamala oil from kamala seed kernels. Petroleum ether extracts only a fraction of the oil from kamala seeds and almost equal quantity of oil containing a higher percentage of kamolenic acid can be extracted from the residual seed cake with ether or benzene. All the oil in the seed can be extracted with ether, ethyl acetate, or benzene[33].

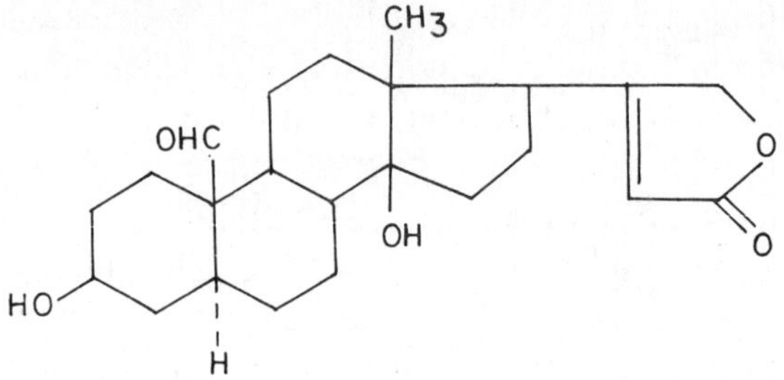

Corotoxigenin L-rhamnoside

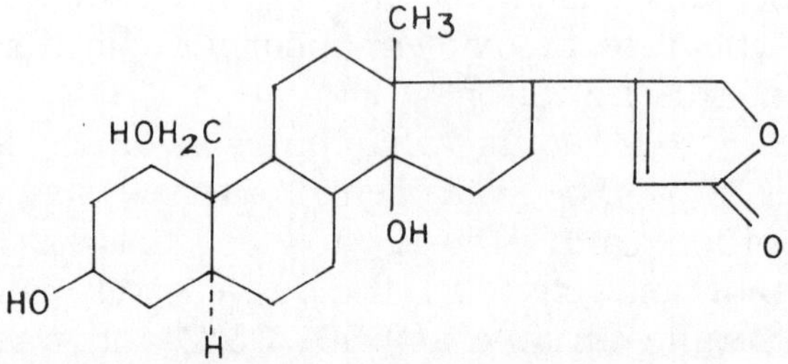

Coroglaucigenin L-rhamnoside

The following table shows the percentage of oil with different solvents and its physical appearance[33]

Table 8.1

	Bhusan *et al*		Puntambekar	
Solvent Used	Oil extracted from Kernels	Physical Appearance	Oil extract from Kernels	Physical Appearance
1. Petroleum ether	43%	viscous liquid	60%	Thick liquid very viscous
2. Benzene	37%	Very Viscous	61%	very viscous
3. Ether	35.1%	viscous liquid	50%	viscous liquid or solid
4. Chloroform	37.2%	Soft solid mass	—	—

Table 8.2 shows the characteristic of Kamala oil determined by Colderwood R.C.*et. al.*[34].

Table 8.2

	Present work	*Aggarwal work*	*Singh & Saran*	*Forest Research Institute*	*Puntam- bekar*
Yield of oil percentage	15-20	About 24	-	-	22-24
Acid value	66.2	6.4	11.3	19.0	5.7
Sap value	203.4	195.0	207.6	170.31	178.3
Iodine value	124.1	166.8	157.3	-	-
Acetyl value	-	16-44	47	49	49
Carbonyl value	-	nil	-	-	26.0
Unsaponifiable percentage	2.6	1.7	1.9	1.8	1.8

Table 8.3 shows the characteristic of the total fatty acids of Kamala oil[35]

Table 8.3

Characteristics	*National Chemical Laboratory*	*Forest Research Institute*
Mean molecular weight	281.2	300.6
Iodine value	182.7	168.0
Carbonyl value	nill	60.0
Diene value	56.6.	58.0

The difference between the carbonyl values of the oil and the total fatty acids determined by Puntambekar as 26 and 60 is surprisingly large. These values for the total raw oil. the refined oil and its total fatty acids have been determined at the National Chemical Laboratory, Pune (India) by the method of Trozzole and Leiber and have been found to be 4.4., 4.2 and 5.5 respectively. The corresponding values determined by the method of Deiths, were nil for all three samples. As pointed out by the first authors, such slight values are caused by the interfering effect or conjugated double bonds even in those compounds which have no carbonyl group.

It was found at the C.S.I.R. Laboratory that the separation of the total kamala oil fatty acids into saturated and unsaturated constituents by the usual lead salt alcohol method was not possible, the iodine value of the soluble and insoluble fraction being 177.0 and 143 respectively. Also some of the acids were polymerized during the treatment. It was however found that if petroleum (40-60) is added to the total fatty acids, an insoluble acid was obtained which melted at 78-79°C after crystallisation from benzene and/or ethyl acetate. When the light petroleum suspension of this acid is irradiated in U.V. Light in presence of traces of iodine it is changed into its β-isomer, melting at 90-91°C. The two isomeric acids have been designated asα and β-Kamolenic acid. Both the acids are unstable and polymerized materials are partially isoluble in chloroform and carbon tetrachloride[35].

The composition of Kamala oil as determined by Bhusan and Wagle, S.S. *et.al.*[36,37].

Percentage of Oil in kernels	Fatty acid composition	
	Saturated	Unsaturated
32%	lauric 0.1%	Oleic 16.5%
	Myristic 2.3%	Linoleic 11.7%
	Palmitic 7.5%	Kamolenic 57.5%
	Stearic 0.5%	

The kamala seed oil can be stablished by keeping it with 5% petroleum ether (40-60°C) for a long time. But this treatment can not be adopted in industry because of highly inflammable nature of petroleum ether. Addition of an antioxidant (e.g. hydroquinone or α-naphthylamine in amount varying from 0.5-1% is therefore necessary if the oil is to be prevented from gelling[38].

Kamala oil extracted from the whole seed with petroleum ether. commercial hexane or benzene is dark brown in colour and can not be used for preparation of pale coloured varnishes and paints. The probable impurities contributing to the decolouration of the oil are kamala dye which remains partly deposited on the outside of the shell. Bleaching of oil by carbon and activated earths was found impracticable due to highly viscous nature and its great susceptibility to heat. Washing of whole seeds with alcohol prior to their grinding and extraction with solvents gives a satisfactory pale coloured oil[39].

The changes occurring in the physical and chemical characteristics of total kamala seed oil and its fractions when heated at 100°, 150° and 200°C in air and in inert atmosphere have been investigated and compared with similar data for tung oil, and it was found that kamala seed oil polymerizes more rapidly than tung oil[40].

Benzene extracted kamala seed oil on alcoholysis with monohydric alcohols such as butyl or amyl alcohol in presence of hydrochloric acid yield modified oil having gelation properties similar to those of tung oil. The addition of more than 60% of other drying oils to kamala seed oil is necessary to give a modified oil of desired gelling quality. The modified oil gave varnishes which were slightly inferior in hardness, drying and other characteristics to those prepared from tung oil[41,42]. The film properties of kamala seed oil and its derivatives can also be improved considerably on modification with toluene di-socyanate (T.D.I.). The modified primer formulated from this has not shown the failure of ckalking, checking or corrosion for a period of one year[43].

The kamolenic acids from kamala seed oil can be hydrogenated to yield 18-hydroxy stearic acid which has been found to be a valuable starting material in the manufacture of perfumery materials and other fine chemicals. The drying property of oil are attributed to the triene conjugated acids, the hydroxy acid and the kamolenic acid (55-60%)[44,45].

The seed cake left after the extraction of oil may be used as manure and it contains moisture (2.86%) protein (8.12%). carbohydrates (35.47%) crude fibres (6.56%) and ash (6.98%). The ash contains phosphate and potash. The cake can be used in combination with sawdust for making insulating boards and cork substitutes. The residual oil in the cake acts as binder[46].

The leaves of kamala tree are used as manure and mature leaves contain 3.29% nitrogen (dry basis) 1.64% calcium the ash (7.83%) is rich in potassium salts[6].

PHARMACOLOGICAL INVESTIGATION ON MALLOTUS PHILIPPINENSIS MUELL. ARG.

The kamala or kamala powder was tested for anthelmintic activity. Aqueous, ethreal and alcoholic extracts were tested against cestodes, trematodes and nematodes and it was found that the drug has taenicidal action both in-vitro and in vivo[47,48].

The purgative activity of drug was tested on rats. One group of 4 rats fasted overnight, was given the suspension of *M. philippinensis* 10 mg/150 gm. rat. Another group of similar rats were fed with gum acacia mucilage in same quantity to serve as control. The faeces were collected on blotting paper and the wet area marked on the paper was measured and it was found that the powder has a significant purgative activity.

The anthelminitic activity of the powder has been investigated in rats naturally infested with *Taenia solium.* The resin in 60 and 120 mg/kg. dose exhibited lethal anthelmintic affect (35.69% and 78.2% respectively) on the population of tape worms[49,50].

Gujral *et. al.*[27] (1960) found that *M. philippinensis* possesses antifertility effects when tested on rats. The active principle was rottlerin.

Many workers also found that powder of fruits reduces fertility in albino rats[51-54].

Gupta *et. al.*[55] (1946) studied that the kamala is used as a coloring agent for hydrogenated vegetable oils and its toxicity was studied on white rats and it was found that there were no histological changes in the structure of liver, kidney, and suprarenals of rats examined at different intervals (one or half month, 3 and 6 month) indicated the absence of toxicity of the drug even when given in fairly high concentration[55].

Extract of fruit was found to possess hypoglycaemic activity when tested on albino rats. A single dose of 250 mg/kg was used and the estimation of sugars was done by the method of Nelson[7]. Ainapure, *et. al.*[56] (1985) found that this drug along with other indigenous drug produces hypoghlycaemia in dogs.

Kamala powder was found to be effective in Hymenolepiasis in childhood 96% patients were cured after a single dosage for 2 days. Besides acting on worms in the intestinal lumen, the drug also acts on the cysticercoid stage lodging in the inestinal villi[57]

The kamala powder at $1:10^3$ temporarily paraliysed the cestode *Taenia hydatigena* in vitro and at $1:10^3$-$1:10^7$, the substance relaxed rat intestine segments and paralysed rabbit intestine segments[58].

Sharma *et. al.*[59] (1979) found that the alcoholic extract of drug in doses of 4 X 10^{21} microgram/ml caused stimulation of guinea pig ileum and it was maximum in dose of 4 X 10^{11} microgram/ml. Further increase in doses caused relaxation of ileum.

References

1. Mehra,P.N.,Bhatnagar,J.K. and Handa,S.S.: Researches in Pharmacognosy Part III-IV, **20**, 294 (1970).
2. Khorana,M.L. and Motiwala D.K.: *Anthelmintic activity of Kamala and its constituents.*: Ind. J. Pharm., **11**(2), 37-43, (1949).
3. Kirtikar, K.R. and Basu, B.D.: Indian Medicinal Plants (edition 2) vol III, 2266-2270 (1975).
4. Shabnam,S.R.: *Medicinal plants of Chamba.*: Ind. For. **90**(1), 50-53, (1964).
5. Gupta,R.: *Survey records of medicinal and aromatic plants of Chamba,*: Ind. For. **90**(1), 458-468, (1964).
6. Wealth of India. Vol. 2, 229-232. C.S.I.R. Publication.
7. Dondrial, R.P.: *Study on Arshina tablet and ointment.* J. Sci. Res. Pl. Med., 6(1-4), 69-72, (1985).
8. Wealth of India, Part III, P. 67. C.S.I.R. Publication.
9. Rao.R.R.: *Medicobotany of some Mysore plants.*: J. Res. Ind. Med. Yoga and Homoeop., **12**(4), 53-58, (1977).
10. Negi, K.S., Tiwari, J.K. and Gaur, R.D.: *Economic Importance of some common trees of Garhwal Himalaya: An ethnobotanical study.*: Ind. J. For., **8**(4), 276-289, (1985).
11. Maithani, B.P.: *Medicinal plants of Western Garhwal:* Khadi Gramodyog, **19**(5), 269-278, (1973).
12. Khan. S.S. and Chaghtai, S.A.: *Ethnobotanical study of plant used for curing skin afflictions:* Ancient Sci. Life, **1**(4), 236-238, (1982).
13. Kapur, S.K. and Sarin, Y.K.: *Economically useful plants of Trikuta Hills:* Ind. J. For., 5(2), 105-110, (1982).

14. Tschrich: As an Handbuckder Pharmakognosie Leipzig Vol III, 27, (1923).
15. McGookin, A., Reed, F.P., and Robertson, A,: J. Chem. Soc., 748, (1937).
16. McGookin, A. Percival, A.B. and Robertson, A.: J. Chem. Soc., 309, (1938).
17. Backhouse T. and Robertson, A.: J. Chem. Soc., 1257, (1939).
18. McGookin, A., Robertson, A. and Tittensor, E.: J. Chem. Soc., 1579 (1939).
19. McGookin, A., Robertson, A. and Tittensor, E.: J. Chem. Soc., 1587, (1939).
20. Narang, K.S., Ray, J.N., and Roy, B. S.: J. Chem. Soc., 1862, (1937).
21. Bakshi, H.S., Jalota, R.S., Narang, K.S and Ray, J.N.: Curr. Sci., 8. 165, (1939)
22. Brockmann, H. and Maier, K.: Ann. Chem., 535, 149, (1938).
23. Brockmann, H. and Maier, K.: Ann. Chem., 541, 53, (1939)
24. Cordillo. G. Marlini, L., Mondelli, R. and Moreschini, L.: Gazz. Chim. Ital. 95, 725, (1965).
25. Crombie, L., Green C.L., Tuck, B. and Whiting, D.A. : J. Chem. Soc., 2265, (1968)
26. Lounasmaa, M, Widen. C.J., Tuff, C.M. and Huhtikangas, A: *On the phloroglucinol derivatives of Mallotus philippinensis* : Planta Med., 28, 13-28, (1975)
27. Gujral, M., Verma, R.D., Sareen, K.N.: *Preliminary observation on the antifertility effect of some indigenous drug;* Ind. J. Med. Res., 48(1), 46-58. (1960)
28. Govindarajan. S.V. and Banerjee, B.N.: *Use of Kamala as an antioxidant of ghee:* Curr. Sci., 8(12). 559-560. (1939).
29. George, J. and Kohil, R.C.: *Nitrogen content of leaves of some Indian trees:* Ind. For., 83(4), 287-288, (1957).
30. Abdul Hamid Khan: *Tannin yielding species, their growth and climate requirement:* Pakist. J. For., 6(2), 78-106, (1956).
31. Bandopadhyay. M., Dhingra, V.K., Mukherjee, S.K.: Paradeshi, N.P., Seshadri, T.R.,: *Triterpenoid and other*

constitutents of M. philippinensis: Phytochem., 11(4), 1511 (1972).

32. Robberts, K.D., Weiss, E. and Reichstein, T.: Helv. Chim. Acta. **46**. 2886, (1963).

33. Gupta S.C., and Aggarwal, J.S.: *Sovents for extraction of oil from kamala seeds:* J. Sci. Indust. Res., **12B**(11). 545, (1953).

34. Colderwood, R.C. and Gustone, F.D.: J. Sci. Food. Agric. 5(8), 382, (1954).

35. Aggarwal, J.S.,: *Kamala seed oil.* J. Sci. Food. Agric. 6(7), 364, (1955).

36. Bhusan, D.: *Non edible oil seeds of forest origin:* Ind. Oil. Seeds J., 3(1), 19-36, (1959).

37. Wagle. S.S. *et. al.:* *Indian non edible oils industry: A techno economic perspective:* Ind. Oilseed. J., 8(3), 198-205, (1964).

38. Kapadia. V.H. and Aggarwal, J.S.: *Stabilization of kamala seed oil:* J. Sci. Industr. Res., 1**4B**(4), 186,(1955).

39. Ojha, V.N., Aggarwal, J.S., and Sharma, P.G.: *Pale coloured fatty oil from kamala seed:* J. Sci. Industr. Res. 15B(9), 551-552, (1956).

40. Ojha. V.N., and Aggarwal, J.S.: *Heat treatment of kamala seed oil:* J. Sci. Industr. Res. **15B**(11), 656-660, (1956).

41. Ojha, V.N., Sharma, P.G., and Aggarwal, J.S.: *Modification of kamala seed oils for varnishes and paints:* J. Sci. Industr. Res., 16A(6), 231-217, (1957).

42. Menon, M.C., Sharma, P.G. and Aggarwal J.S.: *Coating composition from modified kamala seed oil:* J. Sci. Industr. Res. 17A(7), 279-281, (1958).

43. Mishra, J.P., Sivasamban, M.A. and Aggarwal, J.S.: *Polyurethanes from kamala seed oil and its derivatives:* Paintindia, **20**(9), 27-30, (1970).

44. *Utilization of kamala seed, a forest waste product:* Oil and Oilseeds J. **21**(1), 5,(1968).

45. Saxena, M.S. and Aravamudhon, S.: *Oils-interface with paint industry:* Paintindia, **19**(3), 26-29, 31, (1969).

46. Aggarwal, J.S., Ojha, V.N., and Sharma, P.G.: J Sci. Industr. Res. **7B**, 136 (1948).

47. Shrivastava, M.C., Singh, S.W., and Tiwari, J.P.: *Anthelmintic activity of kambila powder:* Ind. J. Med. Res. 55(7), 746-748, (1967)

48. Oliver Bever B. : *Anti-infection therapy with higher plants:* J. Ethano. Pharmacol. 9(1). 1-83, (1983).

49. Verma, P., Gupta, S.S. and Aggarwal, S.K.: *Purgative and anthelmintic activity in Mallotus philippinensis:* Ind. J. Pharmacol., 13(1), 103, (1981).

50. Gupta, S.S. and Verma: P.: *Purgative and anthelmintic effects of M. philippinensis in rats against tape worms.* Ind. J. Physiol. Pharmacol. 28(1), 63-66, (1984).

51. Malhi, B.S, and Trivedi, V.P.: *Vegetable antiferitlity drugs of India:* Quart. J. Crude Drug Res., 12(3), 1922-1928, (1972).

52. Guru, L.V. and Tiwari, P.: *Observation on the antifertility effect of an indigenous compound.:* Nagarajun, 9, 15, (1964).

53. Guru, L.V. and Tiwari, P.: Nagarajan, 2, 211, (1966).

54. Saxena, V.K.: *Antifertility agent of plant origin.:* J. Res. Ind. Med., 8(3), 79-86, (1973).

55. Gupta, J.C. and Chatterjee, M.C.: *Kamala as a colouring agent for hydrogenated vegetable oils: Its toxicity on white rats:* Sci, and Cult., 11(7), 375-377, (1946).

56. Ainapure, S.S.: *Hypoglycaemic activity of an indigenous preparation:* Ind. J. Pharmacol. 17(4) , 238-239. (1985).

57. Dikshit, S.K. and Lalit, O.P.: *Hymenolepiasis in childhood and its treatment by indigenous drugs:* Ind. J. Med. Res., 58(5), 616-621, (1970).

58. Nurtaeva. K.S.: Med. Parazitol, Parazitol. Bolez, 41(6), 741-745, (1972).

59. Sharma, R.D., Tiwari, P.V., Chaturvedi, C. and Pandey, H.S., *Pharmacological studies on M. philppinensis,* Ind. J. Pharm. Sci, **41**(6), 248, (1979).

9
Momordica charantia Linn

Plants have been widely used for various diseases from times immemorial. Many herbal remedies individually or in combination with different formulation such as leaf powder, pastes, decoction, infusion and pills etc. have been recommended in various medical treatises for different ailments. Diabetes is no exception. Indian Materia Medica has also recorded various drug items collected from folklore and traditional practices. But no medicine capable of giving radical cure of diabetes has yet been discovered. Insulin therapy has made great strides in the past five decades but with certain limitation. Recent attention is paid to the study of biochemical modus operandi of diabetic syndrome and connected factors[1].

Although insulin gives best replacement therapy for the juvenile type of disease (it is due to severe deficiency of insulin and leads to tissue wasting, ketosis and ketonurea). While for maturity onset type (less severe and patient retains considerable number of functioning β cells), so in recent years emphasis has been to identify as many plants as possible which could effectively control the disease. Nadkarni's Indian Materia Medica gives the names of 42 plants which are considered to be useful in diabetes. Aiman also tested 35 plants which have been tested clinically for their curative properties in last two decades. Chowdhary and Vohra reviewed the work done on 21 plants for their antidiabetic activity. Israili gives a detailed account of diabetes with reference to Unani System of Medicine and lists the drugs with hypoglycemic (antidiabetic) activity[1].

In the course of literature survey it is found that about 75 Indian plants have been known to possess hypoglycemic activity. Some of these plants are being used by the practitioners of indigenous systems of medicine either singly or in combination with other plants. Ten plants have been studied in detail namely *Allium cepa, Coccinia indica, Ficus bengalensis, F. glomerata, Momordica charantia, Gymnema sylvestre, Scoporia dulcis and Syzygium cumini, Pterocorpus marsupium and Rauwolfia serpentina*[1].

They have been tried on human beings also, Conflicting reports on the hypoglycemic activity of some plants may be due to number of variables such as botanical identity of drug, time and place of collection, mode of administration of drug and type of experimental animal.

Present drug under consideration, *Momordica charantia* commonly called Karela, bitter gourd or balsam pear is widely distributed throughout India.

It is a monoecious climber, Stem is slender pubescent with suborbicular leaves and solitary yellow flowers. Fruits are 5-25 cm long, pendulous, fusiform, beaked and they are ribbed with numerous tubercles. Seeds are brownish, 13-16 cm long, compressed in pulp of fruit. Fruits differ in size, colour, surface characters, habit of growth and period of maturation[2].

Plant is cultivated during warm season from April to June-July. Seeds are sown in line two feet apart on well prepared and manured beds. They are watered twice a week and begin to flower in 30-35 days after sowing. Fruits become ready for collection after 15-20 days[3].

PHYTOCHEMICAL INVESTIGATION OF MOMORDICA CHARANTIA

Analysis of whole fruit shows that it contains moisture, protein, fat, carbohydrate, mineral matter, namely calcium, phosphorus, iron, copper and potassium. Various vitamins like riboflavin, thiamine, ascorbic acid and ascorbegenin (a bound form of ascorbic acid)[4]. Free amino acids are also present in the fruit which include glutamic acid, α-alanine, β-alanine, phenyl alanine, proline, γ-aminobutric acid serine, threonine, pipecoli acid. Green fruit contains luteolin. Presence of free amino acids indicate that fruit contains large amount of proteolytic enzymes[5].

Seeds yield 26.5% clear reddish brown semidrying oil. Oil is edible and mainly composed of a eleostearic acid, linoleic acid, oleic acid and stearic acid[6].

In 1965 Wolfgang[7] reported the presence of a steroidal glycoside and a new stigmastadienol from *Momordica charantia*. Alcoholic extract of the dried fruit gave, chromatographycally homogenous product which is 1:1 mixture of β-sitosterol β-D-glucoside (1) and a new 5,25 - stigmastadiene-3β-ol-β-D-glucoside (II) It was named as charantin.

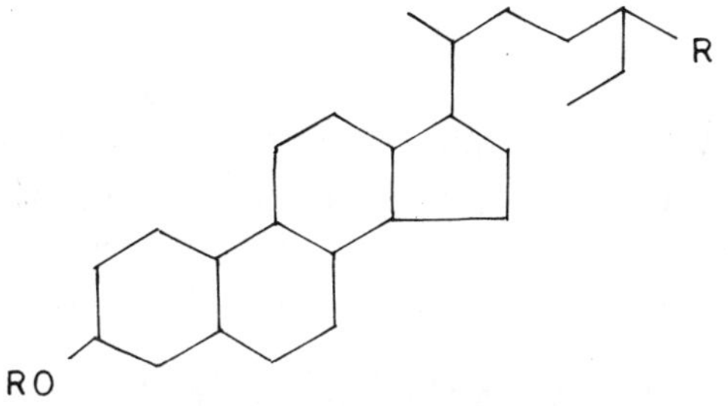

In 1966 Indian scientists Lotlikar[8] and co-workers reported hypoglycemic activity of charantin. Experiment was performed using rabbits. Further in 1966 Wolfgang[9] *et. al.* also reported the presence of two new sterols structure elucidated by means of chemical and spectral evidence as given below: (Fig III, IV)

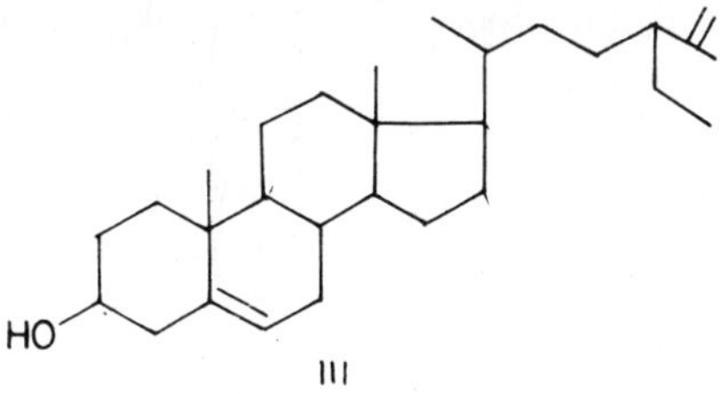

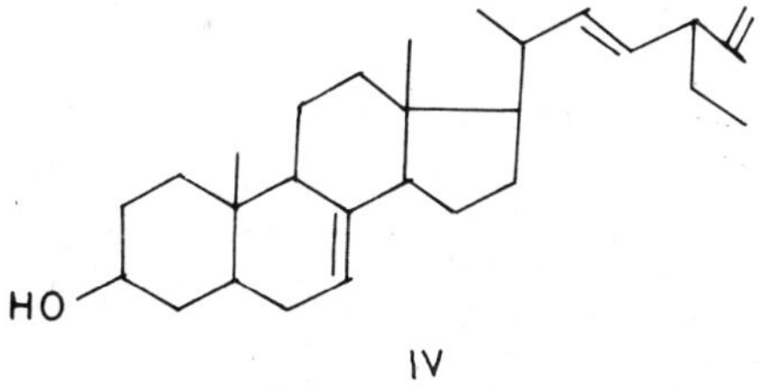

In 1978 Jung[10] *et. al.* toxic and non toxic lectins were isolated from *Momordica charantia.* Both lectins had single poly peptide chain. Lectin named momordin inhibited protein biosynthesis of Ehlirch ascites tumour cells and lectin named momordica agglutinated human O-type blood cells.

Presence of bitter glycosides was already predicted in *Momordica charantia.* Cucurbitacins comprise a group of triterpenes most of which are bitter principles commonly distributed in cucurbitaceae. *Momordica charantia* belonging to family cucurbitaceae tastes bitter and expected to contain cucurbitacins.

Bitter and non bitter cucurbitaions were first reported by Japanese scientists. They were classed as momordicosides. In 1980 Okabe[11] and co-workers isolated and characterised momordicosides A & B, triterpene glycosides. Structure determined on the basis of spectral and chemical evidence.

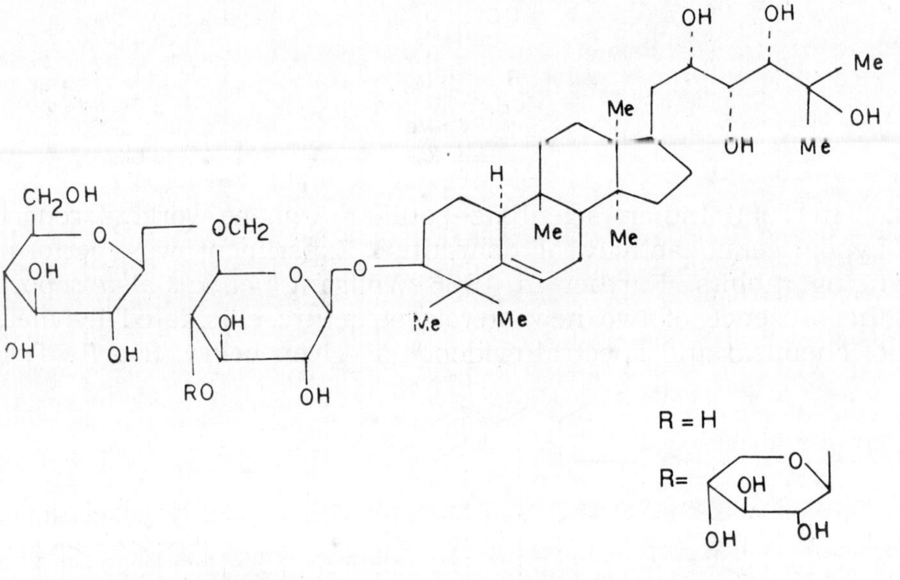

(V) Momordicoside A
(VI) Momordicoside B

In 1981 the same[12] workers reported the presence of three new triterpene glycosides namely momordicosides C VII, D (VIII) and E.

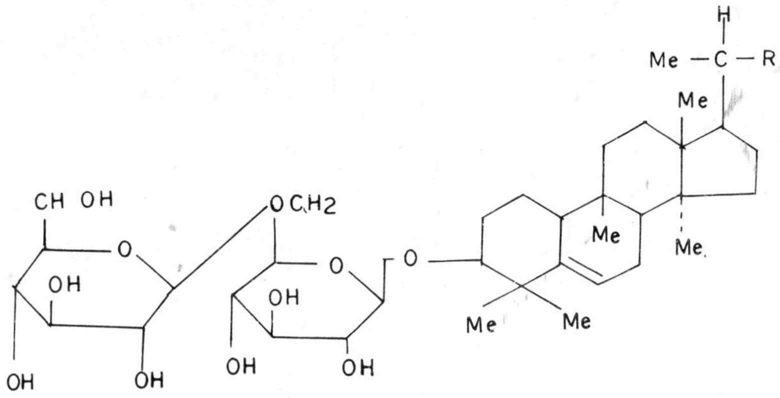

(VII) Momordicoside C $R = CH_2[CH(OH)]_2CMe_2OH$
(VIII) Momordicoside D $R = [CH(OH)]_2CH=CMe_2$

Okabe[13] and co-workers also reported the presence of two bitter momordicosides K & L (IX) and four non bitter momordicorides F_1, F_2, G & I (X). These glycosides were isolated from methanolic extractive of fresh fruits

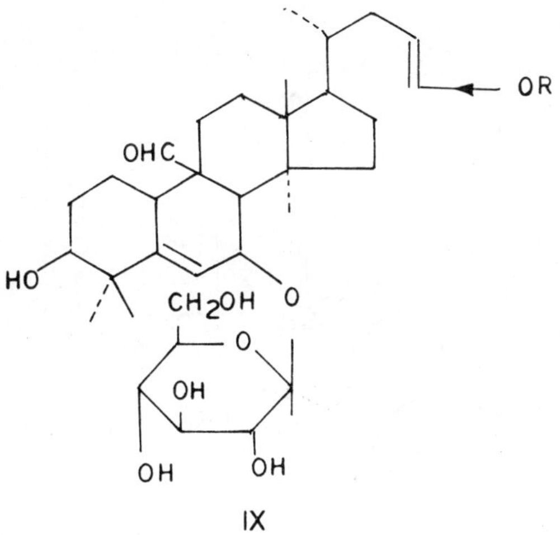

IX

Momordicoside K $R = CH_3$
Momordicoside L $R = H$

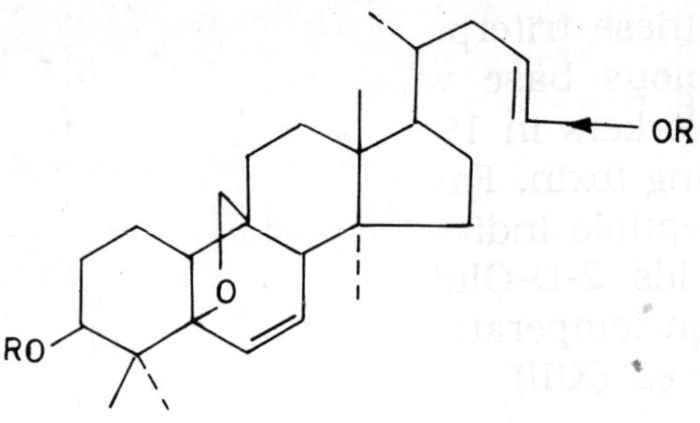

X

Momordicoside F$_1$	R = B-D-glucopyranosyl,	R' = CH$_3$
Momordicoside F$_2$	R = B-D-allopyranosyl,	R' = H
Momordicoside G	R = B-D-allopyranosyl,	R' = CH$_3$
Momordicoside I	R = B-D-glucopyranosyl,	R' = H

These workers[14] further worked on leaves and vines of *Momordica* charantia. They isolated and characterised momordicins I, II, (XI) and III.

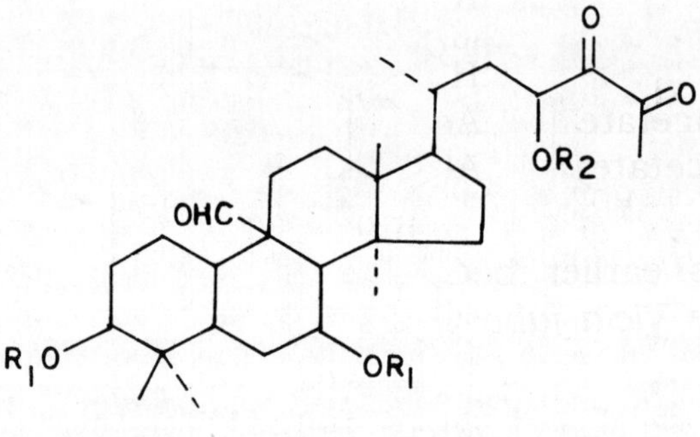

XI

Momordicine I	R$_1$ = H R$_2$ = H
Momordicine II	R$_1$ = H R$_2$ = B-glucopyranosyl

Apart from these triterpenoidal glycosides a glycoside of non protein nitrogenous base was extracted from balsam pear by Dutta and co-workers in 1981. It was named as vicine which is a favism inducing toxin. Favism is an acute haemolytic anaemia in certain susceptible individuals. Vicine with molecular formula $C_{10}H_{16}N_4O_7$ yields 2-D-Glucose on acid hydrolysis, Acetylation of vicine at room temperature afforded penta-acetate and hexa-acetate derivatives (XIII)

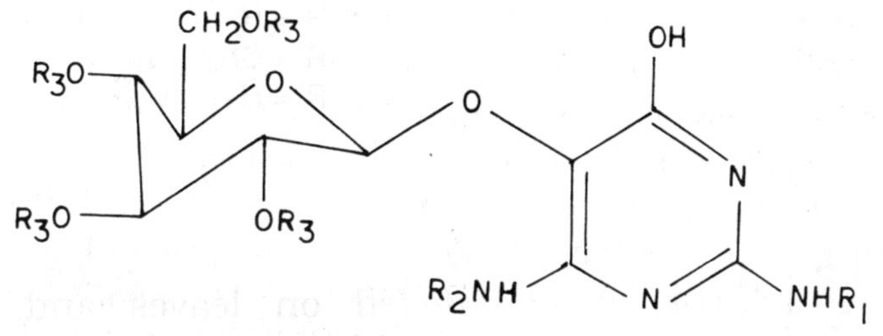

XII

		R_1	R_2	R_3
1.	Vicine	H	H	H
2.	Penta-acetate	Ac	H	H
3.	Hexa-acetate	Ac	Ac	Ac

Vicine[16] has earlier been reported to be present in other plant seeds like *Vicia faba* and *V. sativa.*

PROTEINOUS COMPOUNDS OF M. CHARANTIA

In 1982 Takemoto[17] & co-workers showed that extract from balsam pear preferentially inhibits leukemic lymphocytes due to its cytotoxic effect. This was further supported by Masuho[18] et al who isolated a cytotoxic protein hybrid which has ability to terminate protein synthesis by selective linkage with an antigen present in the target cell. Takemoto & co-workers purified and characterised cytostatic factor, which was isolated by polyacrylamide gel electrophoresis. It was found to be a single protein with molecular weight 11,000.

In 1985 Tun[19] and co-workers reported the presence of an oncostatic agent in bitter gourd. It is a protein with molecular weight of 24,000. A single dose of this protein (50 ug/kg) completely inhibited the growth of Ehrlich ascite carcinoma.

Apart from various toxic proteinous principles, Puspha Khanna in 1979 reported the presence of poly peptide having molecular weight = 6553 containing 17 types of amino acids. This polypeptide was isolated from seeds and tissue culture of *M. charantia* which has been found to be effective hypoglycemic agent when injected subcutaneosly in desert rats, monkeys and human beings. In 1986 Nu[21] & co-workers isolated insulin like molecules resembling insulin in extractability, ability to stimulate lipogenesis and inhibit hormone induced lypolysis. Method involves HCl-ethanol extraction, neutralisation and gel filteration on sephadex G-50, ion exchange chromatography on CM-sepharose.

USES OF MOMORDICA CHARANTIA

Bitter gourd fruit is considered stomachic, carminative used in rheumatism, gout, diseases of liver and spleen. In Ayurvedic system of medicine they have been used as stimulant, blood purifier, laxative and anthelmintic. It has also been used in leprosy, piles and jaundice. Powdered fruit is claimed to be useful in healing wounds. leprous and malignant ulcers[22]. Mhaskar[23] *et. al.* also reported its usefulness in snakebite. The fruit was also found to affect blood pressure & presence of γ-amino butyric acid tyramine and dopamine was reported[24]. Jamwal[25] and co-workers screened bitter gourd for its reputed abortifacient activity. Roots were used for this purpose. In 1978 Dixit[26] and co-workers studied the pharmacological action of fruit extract on testicular function of dog. Chronic administration of the extract for 60 days caused testicular lesions resulting in mass atrophy of spermatogenic elements. It produced infertility state without altering metabolic activity. Further in 1982 Kamboj[27] co-workers observed abortifacient effect of root extract in albino female mice. Pregnant animals aborted fetuses. Drug appears to be effective in all stages of pregnancy and mechanism of action resembles with that of ergot alkaloids.

Maximum work has been done to study hypoglycemic and antidiabetic activity. Pharmacological action was studied on crude fruit extracts, infusions and on the purified compound isolated from seeds.

PHARMACOLOGICAL STUDY ON EXTRACTS & INFUSIONS

In 1941-42[28] infusion of the drug and crude crystalline substance showed marked hypoglycemic action in diabetic rabbits and rats.

In 1960 Sharma[29] and co-workers observed hypoglycemic activity of orally administered Karela juice in normal and diabetic rabbits. Karela juice was given in dose of 2 ml/kg, 4 ml/kg, 6 ml/kg and 12 ml/kg orally after 12 hours of fasting. 6 ml/kg appeared to be optimal dose and maximum fall in blood sugar level was seen after 2 hours. In series of experiments this dose once or twice daily, produced steady fall in blood glucose, both in normal diabetic group. Two female pregnant rabbits died due to uterine haemorrhage proving that drug has some abortifacient action also.

In 1962 Kulkarni[30] and co-workers studied the effect of tolbutamide (an oral antidiabetic agent) on blood sugar level when given with Karela and Jasad Bhasma. Combination of Jasad Bhasma and Karela did not produce any fall in blood sugar level. While if given with tolbutamide, they potentiated the action of latter from fall of 10% to 28% of blood sugar. The Pabrai[31] and co-workers in same year showed that karela fruit juice 10 mg/kg orally once daily produced fall in blood sugar level Gupta[32] showed that extract inhibited hyperglycemia by influencing glucose tolerance in albino rats.

In 1977 Vimladevi[33] and co workers reported the hypoglycemic activity of leaves of *M. charantia*. Preliminary screening for hypoglycemic activity from the ether extract of alcoholic concentrate showed to have equal activity as compared to that of tolbutamide. In 1981 another attempt was made by Akhtar[34] and co-workers to screen the alleged activity of lowering the blood glucose level of alloxan diabetic male albino rats by *M. charantia*. A dose of 0.5 g/kg caused decrease which was maximum at 10 hr. interval. Further in 1982 *Morrison*[35] & co workers used number of plants including, *M. charantia* & *M. balsamina* for screening of antidiabetic property in dogs M. charantia showed significant activity. Samir Yahia[36] worked on various indigenous herbs having antidiabetic property and included *M. charantia* also.

Then in 1984 Chakraborty[37] and co-workers studied various herbal drugs in streptozotocin induced diabetic rats and mentioned the importance of *M. charantia*. Aqueous decoction[38] of the fleshy part of fruit administered orally by stomach tube in rats showed hypoglycemia.

In 1985 Mier[39] & co workers studied the effect of extract of fruit on glucose metabolism and glucose uptake. Fruits at all ripening stages were found to contain two inhibitory compounds, one against hexokinase activity and other against glucose uptake by rat intestinal fragments. Glucose oxidation as measured by CO_2 release by rat tissues is inhibited by *M. charantia* extracts by 50%. Early steps of pentose pathway are also inhibited by the extract.

PHARMACOLOGY OF COMPOUNDS EXTRACTED FROM MOMORDICA CHARANTIA

As earlier reports indicated that isolation and characterisation of antidiabetic hypoglycemic agent was possible from *M. charantia*. So Indian scientist Lotlikar[8] & co-workers studied the effect of charantin (previously isolated by Wolfgang[7] *et. al.*) on fasted rabbits. Intravenous injection of charantin (15 mg/kg) decreased blood sugar level for 4 hours after injection. It appeared to be more potent than tolbutamide in hypoglycemic activity. Cumulative hypoglycemic potency curve was not linear but tended to linear as the dose was increased. Reduced effect of charantin in depancreatised cat indicate pancreatic as well as extrapancreatic action. Charantin (10-25 mg/kg) given orally or intravenously delayed the onset of tremors due to tremorine inhibited sialogogic action of pilocarpine nitrate and exerted antispasmodic activity.

Further other phytochemical studies reveal that charantin is structurally similar to foetidin of *Momordica foetida*. Foetidin produces lowering in blood glucose only in normal rabbits and not in alloxan treated. If on the same analogy it may be hypothesized that fruit contain more than one type of hypoglycemic components. Because the fruit extract caused blood sugar lowering in normal as well as alloxan treated animals.

Allied species of genus *Momordica* have also been considered. These species include :

1. *Momordica angustisepala*
2. *Momordica balsamina* (Linn)
3. *Momordica cochinchinensis* (Spreng)
4. *Momordica cabrei*
5. *Momordica dioica* (Roxb)
6. *Momordica elaterium*
7. *Momordica foetida*
8. *Momordica grosveroni*
9. *Momordica tuberosa* or *Momordica cymbalaria*

PHYTOCHEMISTRY AND PHARMACOLOGY OF ALLIED SPP

Momordica angustisepala[40]: Aqueous extract of root was studied for abortifacient effect in albino female mice. Pregnant animals aborted their fetuses.

Momordica balsamina[41]: It was reported to have anticonvulsant activity in American and African traditional medicine.

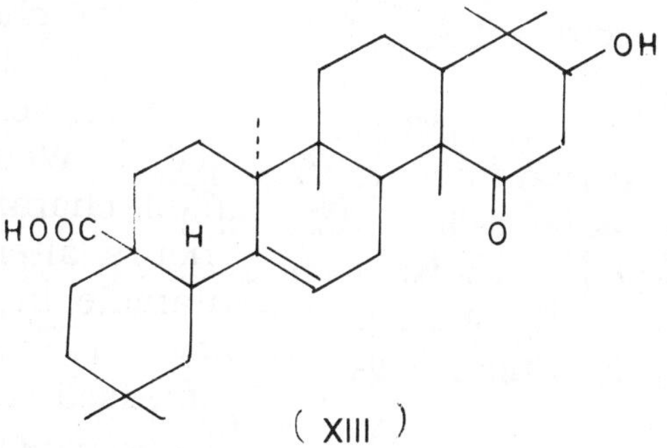

(XIII)

Momordica cochinchinensis : A structure of new triterpene, momordiacid was established in addition to a sterol oleanolic acid and some free amino acids by Murakami[42] *et. al.* Momordic acid (XIII) having empirical formula $C_{30}H_{46}O_4$ and above structure which was established by means of spectral & chemical evidences.

Further in 1971 a saponin gypsogenin glycoside from seeds was extracted by Kobota[43] & co-workers. It potentiated contractile response of guinea pig ileum.

Then in 1985 Iwamoto[44] *et. al.* isolated and characterised root saponin momordin I (XIV), 28-O-β-D glucopyranoside of I is momordin II another related momordin III was also elucidated.

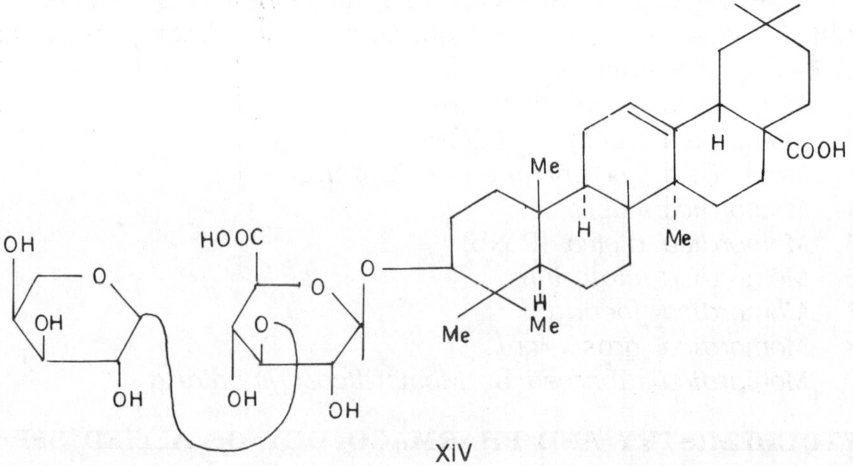

XIV

Momordica cabrei[45] : Aqueous extract of the roots has been traditionally a strong abortifacient. It produces strong spasmodic action when applied to pregnant and non pregnant rat uterine tissues. Active principle appears to be a glycoside hydrolysable elaterase (an enzyme normally hydrolysing cucurbit glycosides).

Momordica dioica[46] : Joshi & co-workers reported antibiotic activity of M. dioica.

Momordica elaterium : It is also called squirting cucumber & it was known to contain elatericin A & B and elaterin by David Lavie[47] (1957-60). Elatericin A (XV) and elatericin B (XVI) have tetracyclic, triterpene structures as given on next page.

They also reported the presence of ecballin A (XVII) having structure as given on next page.

Momordica foetida : From this plant a compound named foetiden was isolated by Nigerian scientists[48] in 1977. It resembles with charantin. It is chromatographically homogenous product consisting of equal parts of β-sitosterol glucoside and 5, 25-stigmastadienee ol-glucoside. Foetidin also lowered blood glucose level of fasted rats. Dose given was 1mg/kg. But unlike charantin

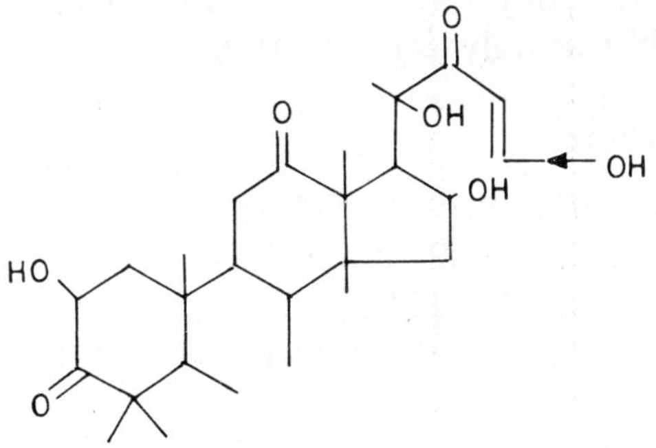

XV

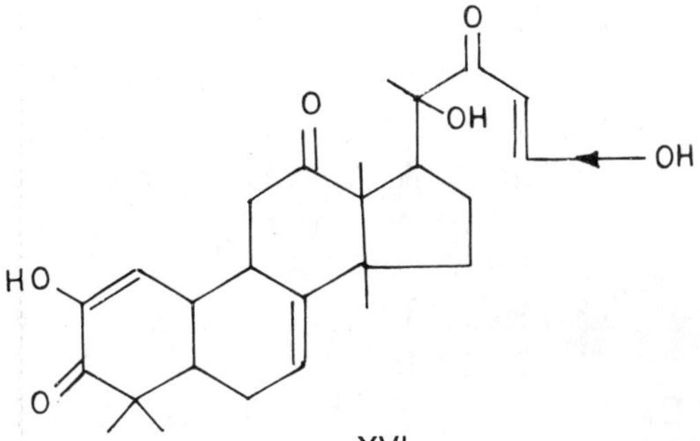

XVI

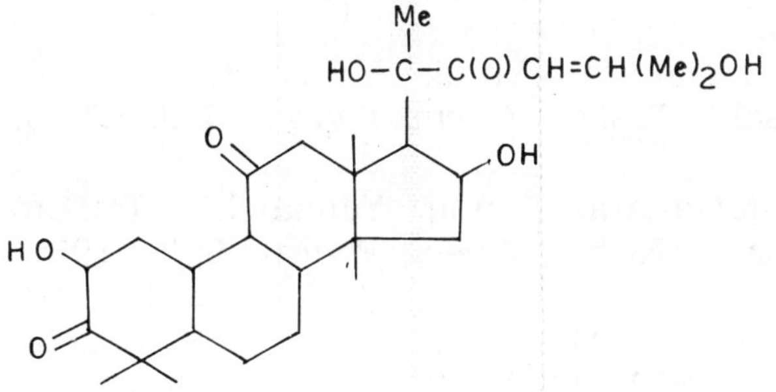

HO—C—C(O) CH=CH (Me)$_2$OH

XVII

it has no antidiabetic action in alloxan treated rats. This may be due to the absence of synergistic compound which may be present in whole fruit. It was also reported to contain a non-quaternary alkaloid[49] and preliminary pharmacological examination indicated that alkaloid possessed strong antinicotinic activity and some antimuscarinic action on isolated smooth muscles.

Momordica grosveroni : It was reported to contain an intense sweetener by Takemoto[50] & co-workers in 1977. Sweet principle was extracted from fruits by hot methanol. Finally the structure was established by these scientists[51] in 1984-85 on the basis of spectral and chemical evidence and they named it as mogroside, a triterpene glycosides. in which the aglycon was mogrol.

References

1. Atal, C.K., Kapoor, B.M., *Cultivatuion and Utilisation of Medicinal Plants,* RRL, Jammu, 1982, Page, 584.
2. Chakravarty, Res. Bot. Surv. India, 1959, 17 (1), 88.
3. Gollan, Firminger, Purewal Farm, Bull. Indian Coun. Agric Res. No. 36, 1957, 93.
4. Pair & Banerjee, *Indian J. Med. Res.* 1956, 44, 749.
5. Rao et al, *J. Sci. Industr.* Res. 1956, 15C, 39
6. Verma & Aggarwal, *J. Indian Chem. Soc.* 1956, 33, 357.
7. Wolfgang, Sucrow (Tech. Univ. Berlin), *Tetrahedron Letters* 1965 (26), 2217.
8. Lotlika, M.M., Rajarama Rao, M.R., *Indian J. Pharm.,* 1966, 28 (5), 129.
9. Wolfgang Sucrow (Tech. Univ. Berlin), *Chem. Ber.,* 1966, 99 (11), 3559.
10. Jung, Yaw, Hori, Mei Jane, Chen, Yon - Chang, *Toxicon,* 1978, 16 (6), 653.
11. Okabe, Hikaru, Miyahara, Yumi, Yamauchi, Tatsuo, Kazumoto, Kawaoaki, Toohio, *Chem. Pharm. Dull.,* 1980, 28(9), 2753.
12. Okabe Hikaru, Miyahara, Yumi, Yamauchi, Tatsuo, Kazumoto, Kawasaki, Toshio, *Chem. Pharm. Bull.,* 1981, 29(6), 1561.
13. Okabe, Hikaru. Yumi. Miyahara, Tatsuo, Yamauchi, *Tetrahedron Letters* 1982, 23(1), 77.
14. Okabe, Hikaru, Mayumi, Yasuda, Masayo, Iwamoto, Tatsuo, Yamauchi, *Chem. Pharm. Bull,* 1984, 32(5), 2044.
15. Dutta P.K.., Chakravarty A.K., Chawdhry U.S., Pakrashi S.C., *Ind. J. Chem.* 1981, 20(B), 669.
16. Devoll. J., Laney. D.M., *J. Chem. Soc.,* 1968, C, 496.
17. Takemoto, Tusunemastu, Nakajima, Tadashi, Zaihara, Shigenobu, Okuhira, Shigery *Kokai* 1977, 7783, 986.
18. Masuho, Hara (Patent) *CA* 1982, (97), 4207.
19. Tun, Tashen, Rivi, Yuyau Kakoi, 1976, 7667, 714.
20. Khanna, P., Jain, S.C. *J. Natural Products,* 1979, 42(6), 684,

21. Nu, T.B., Wong, C.M., Ll, W.W. Yeung, H.W. J. Ethnopharmacology, 1986 15, 107.
22. Sharma et. al., Indian J. Med. Res., 1960, 48, 43 .
23. Mhaskar K.S. & Cacuis J.F., Indian Med. Res. Mem. No. 1931, 19, 54.
24. Durand, E., Ellington P.C., Feng, L.J., Mayne .E., Magnus & Phillip, N. J. Pharm. London, 1962, 14 (9), 562.
25. Jamival, K.S., Anand K.K., Indian J. Pharm, 1962 ? (9), 218.
26. Dixit, V.P., Khanna, P., Bhargava, S.K., Planta Medica, 1978, 34 (3), 280.
27. Kamboj, V.P., & Dhavan, B.N., J. Ethnopharm. 1982, 6(2), 191.
28. Rivera G., Amer. J. Pharm. 1941, 113, 281; 1942, 114 (3), 72.
29. Sharma V.N., Sagoni, R.K., & Arora, R.B. Indian. J. Med. Res. 1960, 48(4), 471.
30. Krishnamurthy, T.R. Antiseptic, 1962, 59(2), 131.
31. Kulkarni, R.D., Gartonde B.B. Indian J. Med, Res. 1962, 24(2), 48.
32. Gupta, S.S. Indian J. Med. Res. 1963, 51, 716.
33. Vimaladevi, M., Venkatesawari, M., Krishna Rao, R.V., Indian J. Pharm 1977, 39(6), 167.
34. Akhtar, M.S., Athar, M.A., Yaquib, M. Planta Medica, 1981, 42(3), 205.
35. Morrison, E.Y., & West, A. W. Indian Med. J. 1982,31(4), 194.
36. Samir Yahia, El Gammal, Hamdard, 1982, 25(1-4), 37.
37. Chakraborty, T. & Poddar, G. J. Instn. Chem. 1984, 56, 20.
38. Gowri Sinnadorai, J. Ethanopharmacology, 1984. II, 223.
39. Meir, P., & Yaniv, Z. Planta Medica 1985, 1, 1216.
40. Aguwa, C.N., Mittal, G.C., J. Ethnopharmacology, 1983, 7(2), 169.
41. Adesina, S.K., Fitoterapia, 1982, 53(5-6), 147.
42. Murakami, T., Nagasawa, M., Itokaw, M., Yachi & Tanaka, K., Tetrahedron Letters, 1966, (42), 5127.
43. Kobota, Kazuchiko, Yakugaku Zasshi, 1971, 91,(2), 174

44. Iwamoto, Masayo, Okabe, Hikeru, Yamauchi, Tatsuo, Tanaka, Tasako, Rokutani, Yoshie, Hara, Shuji, Mahashi, Kuninide, Higuchi, Rijuichi, *Chem. Pharm. Bull.* 1985, 33(1).

45. Organ, A.U. Planta *Medica.* 1972, 21(4), 431-4.

46. Joshi, C.G., Nagar, N.G. *J. Sci. Ind. Res.* 1952, 11B(6), 261.

47. Lavie, D., Shva, Y., Willner, D., Weizmann. J. Am. Chem Soc. 1959, 81, 3058.

48. Marquis, V.O., Adanlawo, T.A., Olaniyi, A.A., Planta *Medica,* 1977, 31(4), 367.

49. Olaniyi, A.A., Marquis, V.O. *J. Pharm.* 1975, 6(3), 117.

50. Takemoto, Tsunemastu, Arihara, Shigenobu, Makajima, Tadashi, Okuhir, Megium, *Kakoi,* 1977, 77, 83.

51. Takemoto, Tsunemastu, Arihara, Shigenobu, Makajima, Tadashi, Okuhir, Megium, *Yokugaku Zasshi,* 1983, 103(11), 1167.

10
Tribulus terrestris Linn

DESCRIPTION OF PLANT

Tribulus is a cosmopolitan genus of twenty species belonging to the family Zygophyllaceae. Three species, viz. Tribulus terrestris, Tribulus cistoides and Tribulus alatus, are of common occurence in India. Among them T. terrestris L. is a trailing plant common in sandy soil, has been described to be of great medicinal value. Tribulus species are usually branching prostrate herbs, usually silky, with white or yellow flowers and spinous or tuberculate fruits.

Among the Indian species, T. terrestris L., which is a trailing plant common in sandy soil throughout India, has been described to be of great medicinal value. It is a reputed drug in Ayurvedic system. It is a procumbant herb. This plant is commonly known in *Hindi*: Chotagokhru,

Gokhru, Gokhuru, in *Arabic* : Bastitaj, Busteyrumi, in *Bengali*: Gorkhuru, in *Burma* : Charratte, Suleanen, in *Chinese* : Chi li, Tsi li Tsi, in *English* Caelthrops, in *French* : Croix de chevalier, Croix de malte, Herbe terrestre, Tribule commune, Tribule terrestre, in *Gujarati* : Betagokhru, Gokharu, Mithagokhru, Nahangokhru, in *Malayalam* : Neringil, Nerimil, in *Marathi* : Gokharu, Lahanagokharu, in *Punjabi* : Bakhra, Bhakhra, Bhukri, Gokhrudesi, in *Sanskrit* : Bahukaantaka, Bhakshataka, Chandadruma, Gokantaka, Gokhura, Gokshura, Gokshuri, Kanta, Kantaphala, In *Sind* : Gokhru, Trikundri, In *South Africa*: Devil's thorn, in *Spanish* : Abrojos, in Tamil : Nerunji.

DISTRIBUTION

Throughout in India upto 11,000 ft. in Kashmir, Ceylon, tropical and subtropical areas, all warm regions of both hemispheres.

MORPHOLOGY OF LEAF

Tribulus terrestris L. (Fig. 10.1 and 10.2) is found to be opposite, abruptly pinnate, one of each pair usually smaller than the other, stipules lanceolate, hairy, leaflets 3-6 pairs, 6-12mm long, oblong, mucronate, base round oblique, Petiole short, pilose. Leaves are diuretic, tonic, increase the menstrual flow, cure gonorrhoea, a decoction is useful as a gargle for mouth troubles and painful gum and reduce inflammation. (Kirtikar and Basu)[1].

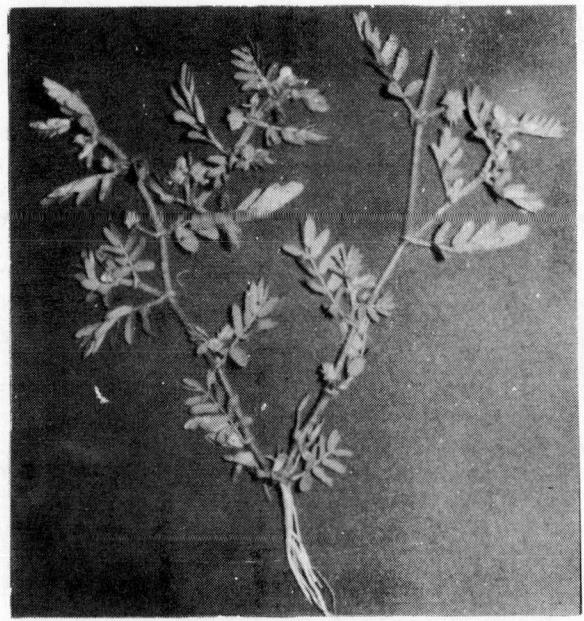

Fig. 10.1 T. terrestris Linn

MORPHOLOGY OF FLOWERS

Flowers axillary or leaf opposed, solitary, pedicles 1.2-2 cm, long, slender hairy. Sepals 6mm. lanceolate, acute, hairy. Petals

1cm long, oblong, hairy. Ovary bristly, style short, stout, stigmatic lobes larger than the diameter of the style (Kirtikar and Basu)[1].

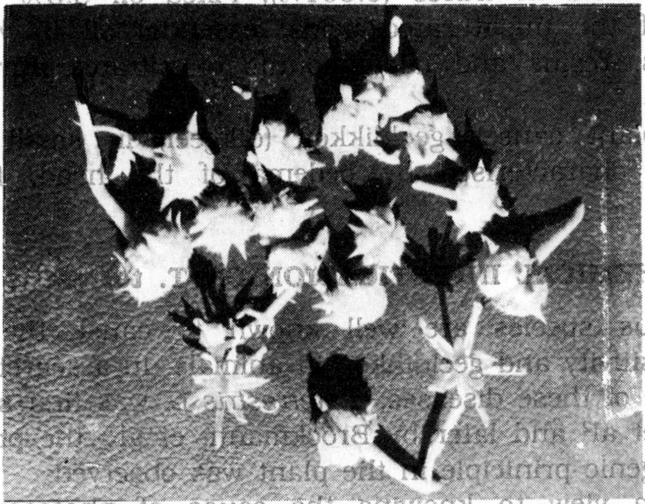

Fig. 10.2 Fruits of T. terrestris Linn

MORPHOLOGY OF FRUITS

Fruit globose, consisting of (usually) five hairy or nearly glabrous, often muriculate, *woodi cocci*, each with two pairs of hard sharp spines, one pair longer than the other. Seeds several in each *cocus*, with transverse partitions between them. They are acidic with a *disagreable* taste, diuretic, removes gravel from the urine and stone in the bladder. They are regarded as cooling, diuretic, tonic and aphrodisiac and are used in the painful micturition, urinary disorders and impotence. In some countries they are reputed tonic and astringent, used for coughs, scabies, anaemia and ophthalmia.

The root is a good stomachic and appetiser, diuretic and carminative. The entire plant, but more particularly the fruits are used in medicines. It was given a good trial in Bright's diseases with dropsy. It was also used, combined with bdellium, in a patient suffering from the gonorrhoeal rheumatism with cystitis. The diuretic property of the drug is due to the presence of large quantities of nitrates present as well as the essential oil which occurs in the seeds. The following substances are found in the fruit:

An alkaloid in traces (0.001%). Fixed oil 3.5% consisting mainly of the unsaturated acids, essential oil in very small quantities, resins and fair amounts of nitrates (Kirtikar and Basu)[1].

The plant causes geeldikkop (dikgeel) in small stock, a condition characterised by oedema of the head, fever and jaundice.

PHYTOCHEMICAL INVESTIGATION ON T. terrestris L.

Tribulus species are well known to cause the diseases photosensitivity and geeldikkop in animals. In a search to know the cause of these diseases, *T. terrestris* L. was first studied by Henrici, et al[2] and later by Brockmann, et al[3]. the presence of an icterogenic priniciple in the plant was observed.

With a view to knowing the cause of photosensitization diseases of domestic animals the plant T. terrestris L. was chemically examined by De Kock, et al[4]. By the hydrolysis of the crude saponins isolated from it, they isolated Diosgenin (A), Ruocogenin (D), Gitogenin (C) and 25-D-Spirosta -3, 5-Diene (D). The hydrolysis of the crude saponins mixture was also effected by a specific enzyme, eletrase (Brown, et al)[5]. In this way, two saponins were isolated, one consisting of a diosgenin aglycone and a sugar chain of rhamnose and glucose and other consisting of a Ruscogenin aglycone and a sugar chain of rhamnose with traces of glucose and possibly arabinose.

The steroidal saponin, diosgenin was also being reported by Kachukhashvili[6]. Also alongwith diosgenin, two other unidentified steroidal saponins were obtained by Kachukhasvili[7]. Steroidal sapogenin, diosgenin, along with the minute quantitiy of the deoxy diosgenin has been identified by Tomova, et al[8] from the Bulgarian variety of the plant. The crystalline sapogenin was being obtained (40%) from the total sapogenin mixture in ether fraction by means of the aluminum oxide column. The other elutes were benzene, benzene-ether (19 : 1), ether and ether-methanol (18 : 2) and finally methanol.

Chemical examination of the dried fruits of T. terrestris L. by Ghatak[9] showed the presence of about 5% of semidrying oil, peroxides, diastase, traces of glucosides, resins, protein and a large amount of inorganic matters. In another examination of the fresh fruits by Ghatak, et al[10] showed the presence of peroxidase whose activity was determined by means of the hydroquinone and hydrogen peroxide. The enzyme was stable below 50°C.

Chromatographic examination of the alakloidal fraction of the herb and seed fraction of T. terrestris L. by Borokowski, et al[11] showed the occurence of *harman* in the herb and *harmine* in the seeds, which are compared with the reference samples. Shah, et al[12] reported the presence of Vitamin C in the whole plant. The total amount of Vitamin C was found to be 78.00-141.66 mg/100 gms.

Shukla, et al[13] have studied the chemical composition and nutritive value of T. terrestris L. and reported it to be rich in proteins and calcium.

Nath, et al[14] reported that the average moisture content in the green plant (post flowering stage) was 65.7%. The percentage of chemical composition on oven-dry bases was crude protein-12.06, ether extract -2.61, crude fibre -27.78, nitrogen free extract -40.83, total carbohydrate -68.61, total ash -16.72, calcium -4.21, and phosphorus -0.245. The plant was shown to be very rich in calcium, calcium phosphorus ratio was very wide (17:1). The dried plant when young (pre-flowering stage) was refused by the animals. However it could be used as a valuable source of feed after the removal of incriminating factors. These incriminating factors can be removed by extracting the dried plant with 5% tartaric acid in 90% alcohol. Three steroidal sapogenins, Diosgenin, Gitogenin and Chlorgenin were isolated by Gheorghiu, et al[15]. Hsu, Chuesn, Chin et al[16] reported the three saponins in the leaf tissue and two in the roots by paper chromatography. Panova, et al[17] reported the presence of Quercetine, D-glucose and L-rhamnose in the leaves of T. terrestris L. These flavonoids were isolated from the ethyl acetate fraction and the identity was confirmed by paper chromotography, mixed melting point and hydrolysis with 5% sulphuric acid. The presence of alkaloids in the the fruits of T. terrestris L. was confirmed by Fong, et al[18]. The aqueous ethanolic extract after freeze drying was taken for preliminary testing of alkaloids, which was finally confirmed by Mayer's reagent (solutions of Potassium Mercuric iodide) and Wagner's reagent.

The two steroidal sapogenins hecogenin (3β -hydroxy-5α-spirostan-12-one) and Neotigogenin (5α 22 α : 25 S-spiroston-3 α -O) from the whole plant of T. terrestris were isolated Purushotaman, et al[19]. They have taken the chloroform extract of the whole plant which upon chromotography over silica gel yielded two compounds A-$C_{27}H_{44}O_3$. Melting point 199-201°C (Vmax 3500 cm-1) and its monoacetate $C_{27}H_{46}O_4$. M.pt 170°C (V_{max} 1725 and 1240 Cm⁻¹). Compounds B- $C_{27}H_{42}O_4$ M.pt. 243°C contains an hydroxyl group (3460 Cm⁻¹) and a six membered ketonic ring (1710 cm⁻¹ and its monoacetate $C_{27}H_{49}O_5$ m.pt -240°C. Hecogenin was also reported by Tomowa, et al[20]. They isolated the steroidal saponins by means of aluminium oxide column. The elutes were Benzene, Benzene-Ether (9:1), Ether-Methanol (9:1, 1:1) and Methanol. Rechromatography over the silica gel and finally by the preparative chromotography.

the compound with m. pt. 243ºC was obtained. The IR spectrum of the compound shows the various absorption bands as 3400 (OH), 1705 (CO), 980, 920 and 860 Cm^{-1}. Diosgenin, β-sitosterol, Stigmasterol and Neotigogenin were also isolated by Mahato, et al[21]. Four samples of T. terrestris L. growing under different climate condition were collected and studied. The highest yield of diosgenin was 0.21% whereas the lowest yield was 0.06% Nag, et al[22] have reported the diosgenin, β-sitosterol and stigmasterol in the root stem and leaves of T. terrestris L.

Free amino acids in the root nodules of T. terrestris L. were qualitatively analysed by Ather, et al[23] using micro-chromatography. Altogther twenty two free amino acids were identified. Glutamic acid, Glutamine, Aspartic acid and Aspargenine being the major amino acids. These amino acids resemble with the amino acids of the leguminous nodules which suggest a chemotaxonomic link between these two major groups of nodulated angiosperms. Other amino acids identified are Cystin, Cysteine, Tryptophan, Serin, Proline, Glycine, Alanine, Valine, Methionine, Leucine, Isoleucine, Tyrosine, Phenylalanine, Amino Butyric Acid, Ornithine, Histidine and Arginine.

Chakravarti, et al*[24] isolated Diosgenin from the weeds of T. terrestris L. Seth, et al[25] reported the Sodium, Potassium and Calcium contents in the fruits of T. terrestris L.

PHARMACOLOGICAL SCREENING

The plant T. terrestris L. is one of the most important ingredients of an Ayurvedic preparation. The drug is diuretic, tonic, aphrodisiac and often used in painful micturition. The freshly expressed juice of the aqueous extract of the whole plant contains inorganic nitrites, mostly potassium nitrite in toxic amounts. It is also used for the treatment of piles, cough, calculi, and leprosy. Pharmacological study on the Indian variety of T. terrestris L. have been carried out by Bose, et al[26]. The minor alkaloidal fraction did not affect the blood pressure of the dog, but depressed the frog heart in situ. It produced inhibition of acetylcholine, induced contraction of isolated intestine of rats, and also of frog rectus muscle and had moderate diuretic effect. The aqueous fraction induced mild hypotension, showed anti-acetylcholine like action on the rat intestine. Its diuretic effect was insignificant. These observations were supported by the results of preliminary clinical trials on selected cases of ascites and edema.

The cardiac action of T. terrestris L. was also studied by Seth, et al[25]. They have reported the cardiac stimulant action of the semipurified water soluble extract of fruits of T. terrestris L. These investigations were carried out on rabbit auricle; cat papillary muscle and on arterial blood pressure of guinea pig. The extract had a potent stimulant effect on the isolated heart muscle in hypodynamic state. An increase in the force of myocardial contraction with a negative chromotropic effect suggested the presence of a glucoside fraction in the extract, Chakraborty, et al27 studied the various pharmacological action and reported that an alcoholic extract of the plant (whole) produced a sharp vasodepression in an anaesthetiised dogs mediated through cholinergic mechanism. It is also some characteristic changes in CNS and carbohydrate metabolism.

In a research news published in Indian Forester[28] (1963), the seeds of the T. terrestris was found to be toxic to the liver of rat. The seeds of the Gokhru was fed to liver, lungs and kidney of a rat for two months. Lungs and kidney on histopathological examinations were found to be normal. Liver, however, showed the extensive metamorphosis of liver cells, Lobular architecture of the liver cells was greatly disturbed. Some of the liver cells had undergone complete narcosis.

Toxicity of T. terrestris was also studied by Sastry[29]. He gave 4 lb of fresh gokhru plant to goats and sheeps and 8 lb of fresh gokhru plant to calves. The temperature, pulse, respriation and body weight of the animals were recorded at the regular intervals. All the animals, were exposed to strong sunlight everyday. Excepting for diarrhoea, observed in calves, all the experimental animals remained healthy and did not exhibit any deleterious effects during the observation period of two months. Fresh juice from 1 kg. of the green plant was administered orally to calf and sheep for a period of eight days. No toxic symptoms were observed.

ANTIMICROBIAL SCREENING

George, et al[30] studied the antibacterial activity of the plant extract (alcoholic extract and aqueous extract) against S. aurens and E. coli and reported that alcoholic and aqueous extracts of leaf are effective against both the organisms, whereas the aqueous extract of seeds was only active against S. aureus. Both alcoholic as well as the aqueous extract of the stem was not showing any antibacterial activity.

Joshi, et al[31] studied the antibacterial activity of 0.9% saline solution extract (treating 15 gm of plantfruit material with 70 ml of 0.9% saline solution for 2-3 minutes and keeping it for one hour) in (1) dilute sulphuric acid (2) Acetate buffer (pH-3.5) (3) Phosphate buffer (pH-9) and (4) Ether, against the S. aureus and E. coli. The extracts in acetate and phosphate buffer were having no activity against these organisms, whereas the dilute sulphuric acid and ether solution extracts were effective against both the organisms.

Dhar, et al[32] reported the antimicrobial activity of the 50% ethanolic extract of the seed and the whole plant (except roots) against the B. subtillis, S. typhi, A. tumefaciens, E. coli and M. tuberculosis.

Sing, et al[33] studied the antibacterial activity of the ethanolic extract (95%) of T. terrestris (fruits) against E. coli by the disc method. They have reported that the plant is completely active against the above said organism.

ANTITUMOUR ACTIVITY

Itokawa, et al[34] reported the antitumour activity of the crude extract of T. terrestris L. The preliminary examination of the antitumor screening was done with sarcoma 180 ascites mice.

References

1. Kirtikar, K.R. and Basu, B.D. Indian Medicinal Plants, I : 420-24, 1975.
2. Henrici and Ondersetepoort. J. Vet. Sci. Animal Ind., 10: 367, 1938. S. African J. Sci. 43:195, 1946.
3. Brockmann and Forsch, U. Fortschr, 19:299, 1943.
4. De Kock, W.T. and Enslin, P.R. Chemical investigations of phososensitization diseases of domestic animals. I. Isolation and Characterization of steroidal sapogenins from T. terrestris L. J.S. African Chem. Inst., 11:33-6, 1958.

5. Brown and De Kock, S. African Ind. Chemist, 13:189, 1959.

6. Kachukhashvili, T.N. Tribulus terrestris as a source of steroidal saponins Farmatsev. Inst., 9:179-89, 1960.

7. Kachukhashivili, T.N. Diosgenin from Tribulus terrestris growing in Georgian S.S.R. Med. Prom. SSSR, 19(3): 46-8, 1965.

8. Tomova, M. & Panova, D. Steroid sapogenins. III. Isolation of diosgenin from T. terrestris L. Farmatsiya (Sofia), 15 (4): 210-14, 1965.

9. Ghatak, N. Chemical examination of the fruits of T. terrestris L. Bull. Acad. Sci. United Provinces Agra and Oudh, India, 2 :163-70, 1933.

10. Ghatak, N. and Giri, K.V. Peroxide from the fruits of T. terrestris L. Bull. Acad. Sci. United Provinces Agra and Oudh, India, 2:171-78, 1933.

11. Borkowski, B. and Lutomaki, J. Chromatographic examination of the alkaloid fraction from the herb and seed of T. terrestris L. Biul. Inst. Roslin Leczinczych., 6:220-7, 1960.

12. Shah, F.H. and Bhatty M.K. Vitamin C contents of some minor fruits and vegetables of West Pakistan-II, Pakist. J. Sci. Res., 14(1): 4-7, 1962.

13. Shukla, K.S. and Ranjhan, S.K. Chemical composition and nutritive value of gokhru. Indian vet. J., 46 (8):715-718, 1969.

14. Nath, K. and Malik, N.S. Chemical composition and nutritive value of T. terrestris Linn. Indian J. Anim Sci., 40 (4): 434-437, 1970.

15. Gheorghiu, A. and Ionescu-Matiu, E. Presence of chlorogenin in T. terrestris L. Stud. Cercet. Biochim., 11 (3) : 269-73, 1968.

16. Hsu. Chuen-Chin, et al. Characterization of the saponin fraction of T. terrestris Linn.Proc. IKla.Acad.Sci., 47:21-4, 1968.

17. Panova, D. and Tomova, M. T. terrestris L. for producing phenol compounds. Farmatsiya (Sofia), 20 (3) : 29-32, 1970.

18. Fong, H.H.S., et al. Alkaloid screening, II. (P.148) Lloydia 35 (2) : 117-149, 1972.

19. Purushothaman, K.K., et al. Occurrence of neotigogenin and hecogenin in T. terrestris Linn. J. Res. Indian Med. Yoga and Homoeop., 11 (1):121-125, 1976.

20. Tomowa, M.P., Botschewa, D.M., Zakin, W.G., and Wulfson, N.S. Steroid saponins and sapogenins. V. Hecogenin from T. terrestris L. Planta med., 32(3) :223-224, 1978.

21. Mahato, S.B., Sahu, N.P., and Pal, B.C. Screening of T. terrestris L. for diosgenin. J. Instn. Chem. (India), 50 (Pt.1): 49-50, 1978.

22. Nag, T.S., Mathur, G.S. and Goyal, S.C. Phytochemical studies of T. terrestris L. Comp. Physiol. Econ l., 4(3) : 157-60, 1979.

23. Athar, M. and Mahmood, A. Qualitative estimation of free amino acids from the root nodules of T. terrestris L. Pakist. J. Bot, 12(1) : 91-96, 1980.

24. Chakravarti, R.N. et al. Isolation of diosgenin from plant Tribulus. Chem. Abstr., (Biochem), 92(6) : 329, abstr. : 91186d, 1980.

25. Seth, S.D. and Jagadeesh, G. Cardiac action of T. terrestris L. Indian J Med. Res., 64(12) : 1821-25, 1976.

26. Bose, B.C., Saifi, A.Q., Vijayvalgiya, R. and Bhatnagar, J.N. Some aspects of chemical and pharmacological studies of T. terrestris L. Indian J. Med. Sci., 17 : 291-3, 1963.

27. Chakraborty, B. and Neogi, N.C. Pharmacological properties of T. terrestris L. Indian J. Pharm. Sci., 40 (2) : 50-52, 1978.

28. Toxicity of gokhru seeds. T. terrestris L. Indian For., 89(12) : 778, 1963.

29. Sastry, M.S. Toxicity of T. terrestris L. Agric. Res, New Delhi, 4(1) : 54, 1964.

30. George, Mariam (Miss), et al Investigations on plant antibiotics J. Sci. Industr. Res., 6B(3) : 42-46, 1947.

31. Joshi, C.G. and Magar, N.G. Antibiotic activity of some Indian medicinal plants. J.Sci. Industr. Res., 11B(6) : 261, 1952.

32. Dhar, M.L. Dhar, M.M., Dhawan, B.N., Mehrotra B.N. and Roy, C., Indian J. Exp. Biol., 6(4) : 232-47, 1968.
33. Singh, R.H., et al. Antibacterial activity of some Ayurvedic drugs J. Res. Indian Med., 9(2) : 66-67, 1974.
34. Itokawa, H., Watandbe, K. and Mihashi, S., Screening test for antitumor activity of crude drugs, *Shoyakugaku Zasshi, 33(2)* : 95-102, 1979.